Multiple Choice Questions in Psychiatry

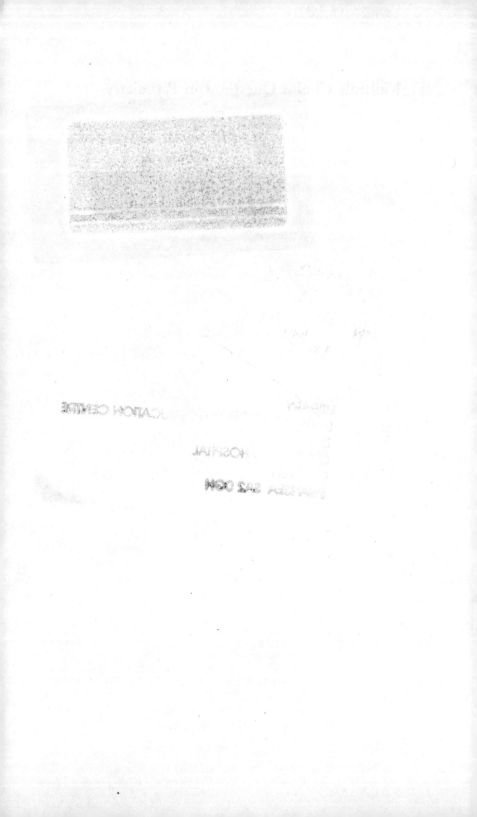

MULTIPLE CHOICE QUESTIONS IN PSYCHIATRY

Chris Ball MRC Psych
Consultant and Senior Lecturer in Old Age Psychiatry,
Lewisham and Guy's Mental Health Trust
and United Medical and Dental Schools,
Division of Psychiatry and Psychology,
Guy's Hospital, London, UK

and

Maurice Lipsedge MPhil FRCP FRC Psych
Consultant and Senior Lecturer in Psychiatry,
Lewisham and Guy's Mental Health Trust
and United Medical and Dental Schools,
Division of Psychiatry and Psychology,
Guy's Hospital, London, UK

A member of the Hodder Headline Group
LONDON • NEW YORK • NEW DELHI

First edition published in Great Britain in 1998
This impression reprined in 2003 by
Arnold, a member of the Hodder Headline Group,
338 Euston Road, London NW1 3BH

Co-published in the United States of America by
Oxford University Press, Inc.,
198 Madison Avenue, New York, NY10016
Oxford is a registered trademark of Oxford University Press

British Library Cataloguing in Publication Data
A catalogue record for this book is available from the British Library

Library of Congress Cataloging-in-Publication Data
A catalog record for this book is available from the Library of Congress

ISBN 0 340 69227 8

Publisher: Georgina Bentliff
Production Editor: Julie Delf
Production Controller: Sarah Kett

Typeset in 9/11 Helvetica by Anneset, Weston-Super-Mare
Printed and bound in India by Replika Press Pvt. Ltd.

CONTENTS

INTRODUCTION

Multiple choice questions are still widely used to assess medical students' knowledge of a subject. They can move through wide areas of knowledge very quickly and are familiar to students. Their weaknesses are well known. Quibbling over the meaning of words and phrases (frequently, often, is associated with) is a time-honoured, post-exam pastime.

This book will not help to develop your MCQ technique very much. We have tried to avoid using these ambiguous phrases as much as possible. In psychiatry, ifs, buts and maybes abound. Because of this we have tried to make our questions relatively straightforward. They cover areas that often come up in exams, but the commentaries take you beyond mere fact. Bald facts are rarely very useful alone but need to be placed in a context. The commentaries will do this. Much, if not all, of the information in the book can be found in the companion volume, *Textbook of Psychiatry*, edited by L. Rees, M. Lipsedge, and C. Ball, and published by Arnold in 1997. Reference between the two books may be useful.

Perhaps the best way to use this book is to work in pairs, late at night over a bottle of wine, taking the stems and questions as a stimulus to talk and learn about the most interesting subject in the whole of medicine.

Chris Ball
Maurice Lipsedge

February 1997,
Sidcup, Kent

Acknowledgements

We would like to thank Joanna Dacosta, Nicola Ng and Brian Thursby-Pelham, U.M.D.S. medical students, for their revisions and comments, and Samantha Bland-Rudderham for her secretarial support.

ACKNOWLEDGMENTS

1 Psychopathology:

   (a) Thought insertion is not a first-rank symptom of schizophrenia
   (b) Erotomania is an overwhelming sexual attraction by a patient towards another person
   (c) Autochthonous delusions appear out of the blue
   (d) A delusional mood is present in psychotic depression
   (e) Delusional perceptions give new meaning to a real object
   (f) *Déjà vu* is not a first-rank symptom of schizophrenia

2 Phobia is characterized by:

   (a) Intense fear of an object, situation or activity which is excessive and disproportionate to the objective danger presented by the object, situation or activity
   (b) The fear is not accompanied by increased activity of the sympathetic branch of the autonomic nervous system (ANS) when the phobic patient imagines the feared object, situation or activity
   (c) The phobic person fears but does not actively avoid the feared object, situation or activity
   (d) The phobic person can be talked out of their fear
   (e) Agoraphobia is a morbid fear of making trouble

1 (a) **False**
   (b) **False**
   (c) **True**
   (d) **False**
   (e) **True**
   (f) **True**

A diagnosis of schizophrenia requires the presence of at least one of the following symptoms for a period of a minimum of 1 month: (a) thought echo, thought withdrawal/insertion, thought broadcasting; (b) delusions of control, influence or passivity or delusional perception; (c) hallucinatory voices giving a running commentary on the person or discussing the person, or hallucinatory voices coming from some part of the body; (d) persistent delusions of other types that are culturally inappropriate and completely impossible.

In the absence of these 'first-rank' symptoms, the diagnosis of schizophrenia requires the presence for at least 1 month of at least two of the following symptoms: persistent hallucinations accompanied by fleeting delusions, incoherence or neologisms, catatonic behaviour or 'negative' symptoms. If the duration is less than 1 month, the diagnosis would be acute schizophrenia-like psychosis.

A diagnosis of schizophrenia should be avoided if there are marked depressive or manic symptoms, unless it is established that the schizophrenia pre-dated the affective disturbance. If there are both schizophrenic and affective symptoms which have evolved together and are present in more or less equal proportions, the diagnosis would be schizoaffective disorder. Before making a diagnosis of schizophrenia, brain disease (such as a tumour), drug intoxication, and epilepsy have to be excluded (World Health Organization 1992: *ICD-10 classification of mental and behavioural disorders*. Geneva: World Health Organization).

2 (a) **True**
   (b) **False**
   (c) **False**
   (d) **False**
   (e) **False**

A phobia is defined as fear of a situation that is out of proportion to its objective danger. The fear can neither be explained nor reasoned away, is largely beyond voluntary control, and leads to avoidance of the feared situation. Phobias have to be distinguished from fear, which is the unpleasant feeling that arises as a normal response to realistic danger (Marks, I. 1987: *Fears, phobias and rituals*. Oxford: Oxford University Press).

3   Parietal lobe lesions are suggested by:

    (a) A loss of ethical standards
    (b) Finger agnosia (an inability to name one's own or the examiner's finger)
    (c) Getting lost in familiar surroundings
    (d) Poor verbal memory
    (e) Left/right disorientation

4   Insight:

    (a) Is an all-or-nothing phenomenon
    (b) Is awareness of one's own mental condition
    (c). Is not important in planning management
    (d) Is retained in psychosis
    (e) Depends only upon the patient agreeing with the doctor about the nature of their condition

3 **(a) False**
  (b) True
  (c) True
  (d) False
  (e) True

Parietal lobe lesions cause visuo-spatial difficulties and topographic disorientation. You can demonstrate visuo-spatial difficulties by requiring the person to copy simple drawings. A history of getting lost in familiar surroundings suggests topographical disorientation. Dominant parietal lobe lesions produce dysphasia, motor apraxia, finger agnosia, dyscalculia, right-left disorientation and agraphia. Non-dominant parietal lesions can produce disturbed appreciation of body image and of external space. There might be dressing dyspraxia. The neurological signs suggestive of parietal lobe lesions include cortical sensory loss causing difficulty in recognizing objects by palpation (astereoagnosis), agraphasthesia (inability to name numbers written on the hand) and visual inattention. Loss of ethical standards is associated with frontal lobe lesions (Lishman, A.W. 1987: *Organic psychiatry*. Oxford: Blackwell Scientific Publications).

4 **(a) False**
  (b) True
  (c) False
  (d) False
  (e) False

Insight is not an all-or-nothing phenomenon and is not merely measured by the person's agreement with their doctor (let's face it, doctors can't even agree amongst themselves at times).
  Insight consists of three dimensions:

  (a) awareness of illness;
  (b) the ability to relabel psychiatric disturbances as abnormal;
  (c) treatment compliance.

  Insight is not retained by those experiencing psychotic illnesses in the sense that they do not believe they are ill, although they may label their experiences as abnormal ('I know this sounds odd but it's true'), and they may agree to take treatment although the reasoning behind this may be far from clear. The degree of insight is therefore very important in planning management. (David, A. A. 1996: Insight and psychosis. *British Journal of Psychiatry* **156**, 798–808).

5   Schneider's first-rank symptoms:

   (a) Occur in up to 20 per cent of manic psychoses
   (b) Are good predictors of outcome
   (c) Include voices talking directly to the person
   (d) Include withdrawal of the sufferer's thoughts
   (e) Include the thoughts of the person being spoken aloud

5 **(a) True**
   (b) False
   (c) False
   (d) True
   (e) True

Schneider's first-rank symptoms of schizophrenia are as follows:

(a) third-person auditory hallucinations;
(b) a running commentary on a person's actions;
(c) voices repeating the person's thoughts aloud;
(d) thought insertion or withdrawal;
(e) thought broadcasting;
(f) delusional perception;
(g) somatic passivity;
(h) outside agencies causing the person's actions or feelings;
(i) primary delusions.

Schneider's first-rank symptoms have become important in the diagnosis of schizophrenia, but they are non-specific when occurring in other disorders, e.g. mania, temporal lobe epilepsy. They also say nothing about the person's prognosis (Crichton, P. 1996: First-rank symptoms or rank-and-file symptoms? *British Journal of Psychiatry* **169**, 537–40).

6   The following strongly support a diagnosis of schizophrenia:

   (a)   Third-person auditory hallucinations
   (b)   Disorientation
   (c)   Visual hallucinations
   (d)   Passivity experiences
   (e)   History of sexual abuse in childhood

6 (a) **True**
   (b) **False**
   (c) **False**
   (d) **True**
   (e) **False**

Third person auditory hallucinations (the experience of hearing two voices conversing about you) and passivity phenomena (the experience that your thoughts, feelings and actions are controlled by an outside agency) are first-rank symptoms of Schizophrenia. Both disorientation and visual hallucinations can be present in people who have schizophrenia, but are highly suggestive of delirium and the cause for this should be energetically sought. Sexual abuse in childhood may precede later mental illness, but not specifically schizophrenia, in addition to delinquency, prostitution, suicide, drug abuse and crime. Adult problems with adjustment are far more common when the biological relationship between the child and the adult perpetrator is close.

The DSM-IV criteria for schizophrenia are as follows.

(a) At least two of the following for 1 month:
   (i)   delusions;
   (ii)   hallucinations;
   (iii) disorganized speech;
   (iv)   grossly disorganized or catatonic behaviour;
   (v)   negative symptoms.
(b) Social/occupational dysfunction.
(c) A disturbance of social/occupational functioning of 6 months or more, including at least 1 month of symptoms from (a).
(d) Schizoaffective and psychotic affective disorder have been excluded.
(e) This disorder is not due to substance misuse or some other medical condition.

7   Type II schizophrenia:

   (a) Responds poorly to neuroleptics
   (b) The person has poor social functioning
   (c) The person has a normal affect
   (d) Has an abrupt onset
   (e) The person is well motivated

8   The following are components of Gerstmann's syndrome:

   (a) Astereognosis (the inability to recognize figures drawn on the palm of the hand)
   (b) Dyscalculia
   (c) Hemisomatagnosia (ignoring one side of the body)
   (d) Right-left disorientation
   (e) Dysgraphia

7 (a) True
   (b) True
   (c) False
   (d) False
   (e) False

Schizophrenia has been divided into Type I and Type II on the basis of the symptoms and signs observed.

Type I	Type II
Delusions	Lack of volition
Hallucinations	Poverty of speech
Thought disorder	Poverty of affect
No neurological signs	Neurological signs
Normal cognition	Cognitive impairment
Normal CT scan	Changes on CT scan
Good response to neuroleptics	Poor response to neuroleptics

Negative symptoms usually develop late in the course of the illness but some may present with these, and this is a poor prognostic sign. Atypical antipsychotics, e.g. Clozapine or Olanzapine, may have some effect upon these symptoms.

8 (a) True
   (b) True
   (c) False
   (d) True
   (e) True

Gerstmann's syndrome occurs when there is damage to the posterior part of the dominant parietal lobe.
   It consists of the following:

   (a) finger agnosia;
   (b) dyscalculia;
   (c) rght-left disorientation;
   (d) dysgraphia.

   It is rare in a pure form, but elements may exist (it is much loved by MCQ setters because of its unambiguous nature).

9 The Amine Hypothesis of Depression is supported by:

   (a) Reserpine causing depression
   (b) The 'cheese reaction' and monoamine oxidase inhibitors (MAOIs)
   (c) Tricyclic antidepressants blocking the reuptake of monoamines
   (d) The prophylactic effect of lithium
   (e) Decreased serotonin (5HT) levels in the brains of those committing suicide

10 The Dopamine Hypothesis of Schizophrenia is supported by:

   (a) Antipsychotics raising the levels of homovanillic acid (HVA) in the cerebro spinal fluid (CSF)
   (b) The dopamine receptor-blocking activity of effective antipsychotics
   (c) Amphetamine may induce a schizophrenia-like illness
   (d) Disulfiram can improve schizophrenia
   (e) Apomorphine can improve schizophrenia

11 Infection of the brain by *Treponema pallidum*:

   (a) Can present with dementia
   (b) Can present with grandiosity
   (c) Can present with depression
   (d) Can present with tabes dorsalis 3–5 years after the primary infection
   (e) Is rarely asymptomatic
   (f) Is always accompanied by neurological signs

9 (a) True
(b) False
(c) True
(d) False
(e) True

The Amine Hypothesis of Depression, crudely stated, says that depressed people have too little serotonergic and adrenergic activity in their brains and manic people have too much. Reserpine (used to treat hypertension) depletes monoamines both peripherally and centrally and leads to depression. Tricyclic antidepressants block the reuptake of monoamines from the synaptic cleft, increasing their activity at the post-synaptic receptor. Most of those who commit suicide have depressive illnesses. Post-mortem studies have shown a reduction in serotonin levels in the brains of those who commit suicide.

10 (a) False
(b) True
(c) True
(d) False
(e) False

The Dopamine Hypothesis of Schizophrenia says that there is overactivity in the dopamine systems of the brain. The effectiveness of traditional neuroleptics (e.g. chlorpromazine and haloperidol) is almost linearly related to their ability to block D_2 receptors. Disulfiram, which inhibits the breakdown of dopamine and dopamine agonists such as apomorphine or L-dopa, leads to worsening of schizophrenic symptoms. Amphetamines cause an outpouring of all monoamines, including dopamine, and may produce an illness indistinguishable from schizophrenia.

11 (a) True
(b) True
(c) True
(d) False
(e) True
(f) False

Syphilitic infection of the brain is now relatively rare in developed countries, but should not be forgotten as a cause of mental disturbances, as it may lie dormant for many years (10–15 years from the primary infection). General paralysis of the insane (GPI) presents either as a dementia, depression or in a grandiose form. Tabes dorsalis is present in about 20 per cent of those with GPI. Tabes dorsalis usually presents 8–12 years after the primary infection, but can wait for as many as 30 years.

12 Pregnancy:

(a) Postpartum psychosis develops in 1 in 500 births
(b) The majority of puerperal psychoses are affective in nature
(c) There is a 50 per cent risk of a further psychosis
(d) There is a 70 per cent risk of psychosis at the next pregnancy
(e) Most non-psychotic depressive illnesses last for less than 1 month

13 Wernicke-Korsakov syndrome may be caused by:

(a) Gastric carcinoma
(b) Hyperemesis
(c) Carbon monoxide poisoning
(d) Tumours of the fourth ventricle
(e) Alcohol abuse

12 **(a) True**
   (b) True
   (c) True
   (d) False
   (e) False

The postpartum psychoses are affective or schizoaffective in nature. In most cases the onset of puerperal psychosis occurs during the first week after delivery, with the incidence rates dropping sharply over the following 2 weeks. The prognosis is generally good, and is better than for matched women suffering from non-puerperal psychoses. The risk of relapse in a subsequent pregnancy is of the order of 20 per cent, and approximately 50 per cent of women will experience a non-puerperal relapse of psychosis at some point. A history of previous affective psychosis (puerperal or non-puerperal) substantially increases the risk of puerperal psychosis to approximately 1 in 5. Primiparous women are most at risk. The main social factor associated with psychotic relapse in at-risk women is a poor marital relationship.

13 **(a) True**
   (b) True
   (c) True
   (d) True
   (e) True

The features of the Wernicke-Korsakov syndrome:

Acute features:

   (a)   drowsiness;
   (b)   poor concentration and short-term memory difficulties;
   (c)   disorientation;
   (d)   ataxia;
   (e)   ophthalmoplegia (6th nerve palsy and nystagmus);
   (f)   peripheral neuropathy.

Chronic features:

   (a)   marked recent memory loss and inability to learn;
   (b)   disorientation in time;
   (c)   confabulation.

The symptoms are caused by damage to the mamillary bodies and medial dorsal nucleus of the thalamus. The commonest cause of this is thiamine deficiency (a, b and e in question 13 above) but other forms of damage (c and d) cause the same syndrome.

14 With treatment the 5-year prognosis for a person with schizophrenia is as follows:

(a) Depends on the family's response to the person
(b) 80 per cent will be back at work
(c) 20 per cent will recover completely
(d) 10 per cent will have committed suicide
(e) 25 per cent will remain in hospital.

15 People with schizophrenia who have large ventricles on CT scan:

(a) Have a good level of premorbid adjustment
(b) Have an increased rate of birth complications
(c) Have normal EEGs
(d) Have the best outcome
(e) Have fewer negative symptoms

14 **(a) True**
   (b) False
   (c) True
   (d) True
   (e) False

The response to treatment in schizophrenia is modified by a number of variables, including the following:

   (a) family response – face-to-face contact with a critical family (high level of expressed emotion (EE) leads to greater rate of relapse);
   (b) cultural background – people do better in the Third World;
   (c) life events – life events whether positive or negative increase the likelihood of relapse;
   (d) social environment – people do poorly if they are in a stressful social situation (e.g. trouble with housing);
   (e) medication – compliance with medication is a major factor; 80 per cent of cases will relapse within 1 year without medication.

Ten per cent go on to commit suicide, whilst 20 per cent have no further episodes. Less than 10 per cent of those who develop schizophrenia have chronic problems that require long-term hospitalization, although many more continue to experience symptoms but can live more independently.

Double-blind comparisons of patients who continue to receive an antipsychotic drug compared with patients who are given a placebo show that over 50 per cent of the placebo group relapse, while only about 20 per cent relapse while receiving an antipsychotic drug (Davis, J. M., Metalon, L., Watanabe, M. D. and Blake, L., 1994: Depot antipsychotic drugs' place and therapy. *Drugs* **47**, 741–73). There is evidence that patients who experience relapses while they are receiving an antipsychotic drug have milder episodes than patients who relapse on no medication.

15 **(a) False**
   (b) True
   (c) False
   (d) False
   (e) False

Large ventricles on CT scan in a person with schizophrenia is a poor prognostic sign. Such people are more likely to be treatment resistant, and tend to have a slow insidious onset of their illness with poor premorbid adjustment. They will suffer from more negative symptoms and require greater levels of support in the community.

16 Poor outcome following electroconvulsive therapy (ECT) is associated with:

    (a) Older age of onset of depression
    (b) Retardation
    (c) Old age
    (d) Neurotic personality traits
    (e) Above-average intelligence

17 Chlorpromazine:

    (a) Exerts its antipsychotic effect through serotonin (5HT) receptors
    (b) May be used in intractable hiccough
    (c) Has less anticholinergic activity than haloperidol
    (d) Causes fewer extrapyramidal side-effects than sulpiride
    (e) Causes photosensitivity

16 (a) False
   (b) False
   (c) False
   (d) True
   (e) False

Useful predictors of response to ECT in depressive illness include the presence of delusions, psychomotor retardation, older age and late onset of depression. Indicators of a poor response include 'neurotic' personality traits, and possibly the presence of recent major adverse life events as the precipitant of the depressive illness.

Contraindications to ECT: ECT should not be given within 3 months of a cerebrovascular accident or a myocardial infarction; high-risk conditions include cardiac arrhythmias, severe cardiovascular disease, obstructive pulmonary disease, severe osteoporosis, cerebral tumours, hydrocephalus and multiple sclerosis. The mortality associated with ECT is approximately 1 per 22 000 treatments. The commonest cause of death is cardiac arrest due to excessive vagal inhibition.

17 (a) False
   (b) True
   (c) False
   (d) False
   (e) True

Chlorpromazine was the first of the effective antipsychotic medications to be introduced to the psychiatrists' pharmacopoeia. It was called Largactil because of its large number of actions. This means that it has been largely superseded by newer drugs, but it remains useful and a 'gold standard'. It does act on serotonin receptors, but its antipsychotic activity is closely related to its ability to block dopamine (D_2) receptors. It has a greater anticholinergic activity than haloperidol, so problems such as dry mouth, constipation and glaucoma are more common. The up side of this is that this increased activity coupled with a lower affinity for D_1 receptors gives fewer extrapyramidal (parkinsonian) side-effects than haloperidol.

Sulpiride, being a relatively selective D_2 antagonist, has even fewer extrapyramidal side-effects than chlorpromazine. Chlorpromazine can be used for intractable hiccough (a particular danger after abdominal surgery), and does cause photosensitivity.

18 Lithium:

   (a) Is ineffective in the prophylaxis of unipolar depression
   (b) Blood levels should be monitored 12 h after the last dose
   (c) May cause tremor
   (d) Can be safely used with a thiazide diuretic
   (e) Is contraindicated in pregnancy

19 Selective serotonin reuptake inhibitors (SSRIs):

   (a) Are contraindicated in patients with cardiac disease
   (b) Can be effective in people suffering from Bulimia Nervosa
   (c) Have cholinergic side-effects
   (d) Fluoxetine (Prozac) has long-lasting active metabolites
   (e) Paroxetine (Seroxat) has a 24-h half-life

18 (a) False
   (b) True
   (c) True
   (d) False
   (e) True

Lithium is ineffective alone in treating unipolar depression, but acts synergistically with antidepressants to treat the illness, and can then be used alone or in combination to prevent relapse. Blood levels should be measured 12 h after the last dose and maintained in the region of 0.6–0.8 mmol/l to achieve the most effective prophylaxis with the minimum chance of side-effects. One of the commonest side-effects, along with gastric disturbance, is tremor, which may occur within the therapeutic range. The use of diuretics with lithium is potentially dangerous, as lithium is excreted by the kidney. Large, unpredictable and dangerous changes in the serum levels of lithium may occur when diuretics are commenced. In the first trimester, lithium can cause cardiac and facial abnormalities in the developing fetus. All women of childbearing age need to have appropriate contraceptive advice before commencing lithium, and the drug should be stopped if they are considering having children.

19 (a) False
   (b) True
   (c) False
   (d) True
   (e) True

One of the great advantages of the selective serotonin reuptake inhibitors (SSRIs) is that they are safe in those with cardiac disease. Tricyclic antidepressants cause cardiac problems both through their quinidine-like activity and through their anticholinergic effects upon the heart, which the SSRIs lack. The tricyclic antidepressants were often stopped because of their unpleasant anticholinergic activity (dry mouth, blurred vision, constipation, etc.), making the SSRIs better tolerated.

Fluoxetine (Prozac) has long-lasting active metabolites, so a long washout period is required before changing the drug to a monoamine oxidase inhibitor (MAOI), whilst paroxetine (Seroxat) has only a short half-life and no active metabolite. There is a recommendation that paroxetine is slowly reduced because of a withdrawal syndrome. Bulimia nervosa can be treated with SSRIs but at a higher dose than is normally required for depression (e.g. 60 mg of fluoxetine, rather than 20 mg as used for depression).

The administration of SSRIs together with MAOIs or with tryptophan (a precursor of 5HT) can cause the serotonin syndrome, which is due to a sudden elevation in 5HT concentration. In the case of the SSRI + MAOI this increase in concentration is due to the inhibition of 5HT elimination. The clinical picture includes restlessness, agitation, nausea, vomiting and diarrhoea followed by hyperthermia, rigidity, hyperreflexia, myoclonus, tremor, hypertension, impairment of consciousness and convulsions. The condition is potentially lethal. Lithium might also enhance the serotonergic effect of an SSRI, causing serotonin syndrome.

20 Benzodiazepines:

    (a) Require regular blood assays
    (b) Should only be prescribed for a short course
    (c) May exacerbate the effects of alcohol
    (d) Are a common cause of death if taken in overdose
    (e) May impair ability to drive a car safely

21 The following drugs may interfere with sexual functioning:

    (a) Beta blockers
    (b) Benzodiazepines
    (c) Haloperidol
    (d) Sodium Valproate
    (e) Ampicillin

20 **(a) False**
(b) True
(c) True
(d) False
(e) True

Benzodiazepines are highly effective anxiolytics and hypnotics, but they are highly addictive and tolerance can develop. They must only be given for short courses to avoid these problems.

Benzodiazepines are indicated for the short-term relief (2 to 4 weeks only) of symptoms of anxiety or insomnia that are severe, disabling, or which subject the individual to unacceptable distress. There is no therapeutic range that should be aimed for, and blood assays are of no value in clinical practice. Benzodiazepines are centrally acting depressants, as is alcohol, so they may exacerbate the effects of alcohol. Whilst they are relatively safe in overdose when taken alone, in combination with alcohol they are lethal. People with COAD (Chronic Obstructive Airway Disease) and low respiratory drive are at particular risk. The effects of benzodiazepines can be reversed by using Flumanazil. As they are centrally acting depressants, reaction times are lengthened, and this can make driving and the operating of machinery dangerous.

21 **(a) True**
(b) True
(c) True
(d) False
(e) False

An important enquiry in any person presenting with sexual dysfunction is a drug history. Phenothiazines and butyrophenones cause loss of libido. This might be due to dopamine blockade, hyperprolactinaemia or other hormonal effects. Tricyclic antidepressants cause erectile dysfunction. The mechanism may be alpha-adrenoceptor blockade. Ejaculatory failure can be caused by Thioridazine, and to a lesser extent, by other neuroleptics, due to alpha-adrenoceptor blockade or anticholinergic action. Phenothiazines and both tricyclic and SSRI antidepressants can cause anorgasmia. Priapism can be a side-effect of Trazodone.

22 Exhibitionism:

   (a) Few exhibitionists are married
   (b) Exhibitionists frequently go on to commit more serious sexual assaults
   (c) It is one of the commonest sexual offences
   (d) It may be a reaction to stress
   (e) The exhibitionist always exposes an erect penis

23 The following are associated with daytime drowsiness:

   (a) Narcolepsy
   (b) Kleine-Levin syndrome
   (c) Sleep apnoea
   (d) Autism
   (e) Seasonal affective disorder

22 (a) False
   (b) False
   (c) True
   (d) True
   (e) False

Exhibitionists have been classified into two types.

(a) Those of the first type tend to expose at times of stress or distress with a flaccid penis, and are frequently married, do not go on to commit more serious offences, feel remorse, and do not reoffend.
(b) Those of the second type expose with an erect penis, do so in order to gain excitement from and the reaction of those exposed to, and masturbate following the exposure. They are more likely to repeat the act, experiencing no guilt or feelings for the person they have exposed themselves to.

23 (a) True
   (b) True
   (c) True
   (d) False
   (e) True

Sleep disorders have been divided into DIMS (Disorders of Initiation and Maintenance of Sleep) and DOES (Disorders of Excessive Somnolence).

The characteristic features of narcolepsy include frequent daytime naps, cataplexy, sleep paralysis, hypnagogic hallucinations, sleep-onset REM periods, very short latency, daytime sub-wakefulness, positive family history in up to 50 per cent HLA antigen DR_2. Cataplexy is characterized by loss of muscle tone, triggered by a sudden emotion. Catalepsy is a form of narcolepsy in which the person suddenly drops off to sleep in an unpredictable manner. They lose their muscle tone and fall to the floor. They can be treated with tricyclic antidepressants to reduce the frequency of attacks and amphetamines to prolong the periods of wakefulness.

The Kleine-Levin syndrome is an uncommon disorder characterized by episodic hypersomnolence, excessive eating, irritability and hypersexuality. Each attack lasts for about a week with the patient sleeping for about 20 hours in each 24.

The Pickweakean syndrome is a form of obstructive sleep apnoea with obesity, CO_2 retention and diminished ventilatory drive to increase in pCO_2. Treatment involves avoiding alcohol, losing weight and stopping smoking. Some people require positve-pressure nasal airways in order to keep the airway open.

In seasonal affective disorder, winter depression is accompanied by hypersomnia, hyperhagia, anergia, carbohydrate craving and weight gain. Depressions usually end by March and may be follwed by hypomania, mania or normal mood in the spring and summer (Parkes, J. D. *Sleep and its Disorders*, 1985. London: W. B. Saunders).

24 Features of LSD abuse include:

   (a) Tachycardia
   (b) Synaesthesia
   (c) Peripheral neuropathy
   (d) Formication
   (e) Dilated pupils

25 The following suggest pseudodementia rather than dementia:

   (a) Catastrophic response
   (b) Short history of cognitive defects
   (c) 'Don't know' answers
   (d) Subject complaining of memory impairment
   (e) Dressing dyspraxia

24 (a) True
   (b) True
   (c) False
   (d) False
   (e) True

Those who take LSD experience a wide range of sensory distortions and delusional ideas. Physical signs of general arousal such as tachycardia and dilated pupils are seen. In addition to hallucinations, they may experience one sensory modality as another (synaesthesia), e.g. colours as sounds. Formication is the feeling of having insects under the skin, and is classically associated with cocaine use (cocaine bug).

25 (a) False
   (b) True
   (c) True
   (d) True
   (e) False

It is important to distinguish illnesses which might present in a dementia-like way (pseudodementia), as they have possibilities for treatment which are not yet available for most forms of dementia. Depression is the illness most commonly mistaken for dementia. The history of cognitive problems is usually short, with depressive symptoms coming before cognitive ones. There is often a previous history of depression, and an informant will not describe the sufferer as having problems getting their clothes on in the right order or round the right way (dressing dyspraxia). A person with pseudodementia is likely to complain of memory problems, whilst a person with dementia may not. When asking questions, the person with pseudodementia will answer 'don't know' to questions and make no attempt to find the right answer, whereas a person with dementia will often confabulate and answer the question wrongly. Neurological signs are uncommon in those with pseudodementia, whilst most dementing illnesses are accompanied by signs, which are sometimes very subtle.

26 The following is true of depression in the elderly:

   (a) One in five remain chronically depressed
   (b) 30 per cent die within 6 years
   (c) Men have a worse prognosis than women
   (d) First episode over the age of 70 years is associated with a worse prognosis
   (e) Physical illness has no impact on the prognosis

27 Normal pressure hydrocephalus:

   (a) Presents with an affective disorder
   (b) Incontinence is common
   (c) If treated early is reversible
   (d) CT scanning does not help the diagnosis
   (e) The patient walks normally

26 (a) True
   (b) True
   (c) True
   (d) True
   (e) False

There has been much discussion of the prognosis of depression in the elderly. Definitions of outcome vary greatly between studies, as does the treatment that these people receive. However, one in five (20 per cent) will remain chronically depressed even if their depression is recognized and treated. One third are dead within 6 years. This number is greater than you would expect for a similar group of elders who are not depressed. Depression is associated with physical illness, but there is still an excess mortality when this has been controlled for. Those over 70 years of age appear to have a worse prognosis than younger patients, and men fare worse than women. Despite this apparently bleak picture, it is important to recognize and adequately treat depression in the elderly, as there is no way of predicting who will respond to interventions (psychological, social or pharmacological) and who will not.

27 (a) False
   (b) True
   (c) True
   (d) False
   (e) False

The importance of recognizing normal pressure hydrocephalus is that the collection of CSF within the brain can be drained using a shunt, and the development of dementia arrested or even reversed.

Normal pressure hydrocephalus presents with a classic triad of:

(a) dementia;
(b) incontinence;
(c) gait disturbance.

All of these symptoms are common in the elderly, and so a high index of suspicion must be maintained. The CT scan has a classic appearance of huge ventricles with the brain tissue pushed up against the skull. In many cases of hydrocephalus no cause can be established, but there may be a history of subarachnoid haemorrhage, head injury or meningitis, which causes organization of adhesions in the basal cisterns (Lishman, W. A. 1987: *Organic psychiatry*, 2nd edn. Oxford: Blackwell Scientific Publications).

28 Hallucinations:

    (a) Occur only in the mentally ill
    (b) Are misinterpretations of external stimuli
    (c) Auditory hallucinations in the third person are particularly associated with schizophrenia
    (d) In the visual modality suggest an organic cause
    (e) Occur in 50 per cent of bereaved people

29 Obsessional rituals (compulsions) generally:

    (a) Are recognized as senseless by the individual
    (b) Are performed in response to hallucinatory commands
    (c) Are not resisted
    (d) Rarely involve checking
    (e) Occur in post-traumatic stress disorder

28 **(a) False**
   (b) False
   (c) True
   (d) True
   (e) True

Hallucinations (perceptions in the absence of external stimuli) do not only occur in the mentally ill. It is a common experience to believe that your name has been called in a crowd, and for bereaved people to see the person who has just died. These people often fear that they are going mad and need only to be reassured that their experiences are normal.

Misinterpretations of external stimuli are illusions.

Third-person auditory hallucinations are one of Schneider's first-rank symptoms and are important in the diagnosis of schizophrenia.

The presence of visual hallucinations should raise the possibility of an organic cause. They can occur both in depression and in schizophrenia, but should be regarded as organic until proved otherwise.

29 **(a) True**
   (b) False
   (c) False
   (d) False
   (e) False

Obsessional rituals are actions that a person feels compelled to carry out. They come unbidden into the person's mind and are regarded as senseless. For some patients performing the rituals relieves anxiety, but for others it has the opposite effect. Compulsive rituals are for the most part resisted but over time some patients no longer fight the compulsion and give in to it. Checking, washing, cleaning and counting are among the most common rituals, and are often repeated a 'magical' number of times. A ritual may serve to 'cancel out' an obsession such as a repetitive blasphemous, obscene or sadistic thought.

30 Somatic symptoms of anxiety include:

    (a) Constipation
    (b) Tinnitus
    (c) Carpopedal spasm
    (d) Pallor
    (e) Tremor

31 Alcohol dependence:

    (a) Is suggested by a mean corpuscular volume (MCV) of 90
    (b) Is suggested by an irregular drinking pattern
    (c) Is suggested by an altered tolerance of alcohol
    (d) Can be recognized by use of the CAGE questionnaire
    (e) More than 15 units of alcohol a week for a man represents an unsafe level of drinking

30 (a) False
   (b) True
   (c) True
   (d) True
   (e) True

In addition to the cognitive symptoms of anxiety (apprehensiveness, terror, fear of death, derealization, etc.) there are a large number of somatic symptoms which are often ascribed to physical illness. These include:

(a) Cardiac symptoms — palpitations, pounding in the chest, tachycardia;

(b) Pulmonary symptoms — shortness of breath, choking, hyperventilation;

(c) Abdominal symptoms — 'butterflies', nausea, frequent and precipitant bowel action;

(d) Urinary symptoms — frequency;

(e) Neurological symptoms — headaches, dizziness, carpopedal spasm;

(f) Autonomic symptoms — flushes.

31 (a) False
   (b) False
   (c) True
   (d) True
   (e) False

An elevated gamma GT is found in 80 per cent of problem drinkers, and a raised MCV is found in about 60 per cent. The normal range for the MCV is 80–96. Most people who are addicted to alcohol drink in a regular way and have an altered tolerance to alcohol. Initially the tolerance rises, but as their liver and brain become damaged the tolerance to alcohol declines.

The CAGE questionnaire consists of the following:

C Have you ever thought that you should **C**ut down on your drinking?

A Have people ever **A**nnoyed you by criticizing your drinking?

G Have you ever felt **G**uilty about your drinking?

E Do you ever have an **E**ye-opener?

This questionnaire is a useful screening instrument for the identification of problem drinkers.

32 The following make a diagnosis of delirium more likely than dementia:

   (a) Preserved sleep-wake cycle
   (b) Abrupt onset
   (c) Visual hallucinations
   (d) Variability in cognitive testing
   (e) Rapidly changing behaviour

32 (a) **False**
   (b) **True**
   (c) **True**
   (d) **True**
   (e) **True**

The diagnostic features of delirium include:

(a) impairment of consciousness and attention;
(b) perceptual distortions and illusions;
(c) hallucinations (especially visual);
(d) impairment of immediate recall and of recent memory with relatively intact remote memory;
(e) rapid fluctuations of psychomotor activity;
(f) disturbance of sleep-wakefulness cycle with daytime drowsiness and nocturnal exacerbation of symptoms;
(g) disturbance of affect, including anxiety, fear, irritability or depression.

	Dementia	Delirium
Sleep-wake cycle	Preserved	Disrupted
Onset	Gradual	Abrupt
Visual hallucinations	Unusual	Common
Cognitive testing	Slow decline	Rapid fluctuations
Behaviour	Stable	Rapid fluctuations

It is important to make a diagnosis of delirium because it has an underlying medical problem producing the confusion, which can be treated and the person restored to their former level of functioning. It is often difficult to diagnose this in people who suffer from dementia, but rapid changes of mental state and behaviour or the development of new symptoms (e.g. visual hallucinations) should suggest the possibility of a delirium.

33 The prognosis of depression:

(a) Is worse for the elderly
(b) Is worse for men
(c) Is better for the lower social classes
(d) Is better for psychotic depression
(e) At least 50 per cent of cases will relapse eventually

33 (a) True
   (b) True
   (c) False
   (d) False
   (e) True

Depressive illness very frequently resolves, but despite very long periods between episodes 50 per cent of unipolar depressives will experience a recurrence (the recurrence rate in bipolar disorder is even higher). The prognosis appears to be worse for men and those in lower social classes. It would appear that those who experience low-grade but disabling depressions are at high risk that this will become chronic and difficult to treat either psychologically or pharmacologically. Those with psychotic illnesses of a more overtly biological nature find that discrete episodes are often treatable by biological means, with long periods of good health between the episodes.

Maintenance treatment should be considered if a person has two or more depressive episodes during a 2-year period, especially those with an onset of depression after the age of 50 years, who are at higher risk for relapse.

Maintenance treatment with an antidepressant using the same dosage as during the acute episode significantly reduces the relapse rate. Lithium is also an effective maintenance treatment for unipolar disorder, but the side-effect profile renders it less suitable for maintenance therapy in this condition, whereas it is strongly indicated in bipolar affective disorder.

34 The following disorders are associated with depression:

(a) Hypothyroidism
(b) Addison's disease
(c) Phaeochromocytoma
(d) Pellagra
(e) Cushing's syndrome

34 (a) True
   (b) True
   (c) False
   (d) True
   (e) True

When making a diagnosis of depression it is important to consider the possibility that there is an underlying physical cause. If this is not recognized, it is unlikely that the depression will respond to treatment. Even if the underlying medical problem is resolved, the depression may require adequate treatment in its own right.

Hypothyroidism is the commonest organic cause of depression, but in addition to those mentioned above, iatrogenic causes (especially drugs) must be considered (reserpine, alpha methyl dopa, L-dopa, beta blockers, calcium antagonists, oral contraceptives, corticosteriods). Other organic causes include hyperparathyroidism, anaemia, post-infective states (influenza, glandular fever and brucellosis) and neurological disorders including Parkinson's disease, multiple sclerosis, cerebral systemic lupus erythematosus and intracranial tumours.

In patients with a physical illness, somatic symptoms such as loss of appetite and weight, disturbed sleep and lack of energy are unreliable indexes of a possible associated depressive illness. The doctor has to rely on affective rather than physical symptoms, and should concentrate on social withdrawal, a low mood that is not reactive to environmental events, anhedonia, morning depression, feelings of helplessness, hopelessness, worthlessness, guilt and the idea that the illness is a punishment.

Creed and Guthrie (1996) provide a useful way of classifying physical illnesses which might lead to psychological complications, based on both their time-course and whether they are systemic or cerebral.

Table 1   Examples of physical illness leading to psychological complications

	Acute	Chronic
Intracranial: generalized	Encephalitis	General paralysis of the insane (GPI) Normal pressure hydrocephalus
Intracranial: focal	Temporal lobe epilepsy	Tumour Cerebral abscess
Extracranial	Any acute infection, endocrine abnormality, etc.	Thyroid disease Cancer (e.g. carcinoma of the pancreas might present as depression)

Creed, F. and Gutherie, E. (1996: Classification of psychiatric disorders. In *Liaison Psychiatry*. London: Royal College of Psychiatrists, 67).

35 Completed suicide:

    (a) The rates are higher in men
    (b) 70 per cent suffer from depressive illnesses
    (c) Living alone increases the risk
    (d) Previous failed suicide attempt decreases the risks
    (e) Incidence is highest in those who have never married

36 Life events:

    (a) Women have higher levels of life events prior to developing depression than do men
    (b) Life events involving threat lead to anxiety rather than depression
    (c) Only loss or threat events precede relapse in schizophrenia
    (d) Having a job increases the impact of life events
    (e) Having no confidence increases the impact of life events

35 **(a) True**
   (b) True
   (c) True
   (d) False
   (e) False

Completed suicide occurs in about 15 per cent of people with bipolar affective disorder and in about 10 per cent of people with schizophrenia. There is also a statistical association with alcoholism. The commonest mode of suicide for men is carbon monoxide poisoning from car exhaust fumes, and for women the commonest method is an overdose of drugs, generally analgesics or antidepressants. ·

Most completed suicides have been planned, and many suicides have given warning of their intentions. About a sixth of people who commit suicide leave a note. Suicide is twice as common in men as in women, and rates are higher in divorcees than in married people.

Suicide rates are higher among professional people and unskilled workers. The rate of suicide among younger men has been rising over the past 20 years.

36 **(a) True**
   (b) True
   (c) False
   (d) False
   (e) True

In order to establish that life events cause psychiatric disorder it is necessary:

- (a) to demonstrate a statistical correlation between the life events and the onset of psychiatric disorder;
- (b) to exclude the possibility that the early stages of the illness itself have not in themselves caused life events (e.g. psychotic symptoms leading to lack of productivity, resulting in job loss);
- (c) it is desirable to assess both the severity of life events and their individual meaning. It is helpful to divide events into those which represent a threat and those which signify loss.

Men are less vulnerable to the impact of life events than women. Those who have stable relationships and jobs are further cushioned. For those who have no close confidant and no job it is harder to deal with life events. Women with three or more young children are also at greater risk. Events that are threatening, e.g. a physical illness, tend to lead to anxiety rather than depression, which happens after loss events, e.g. a bereavement. People with schizophrenia react poorly to almost any changes in their life circumstances even positive ones.

37 Head injury:

(a) Post-traumatic amnesia is a good prognostic indicator
(b) Epilepsy develops in 20 per cent of cases of closed head injuries
(c) Post-concussion syndrome is rare
(d) The prognosis is worse with penetrating injuries
(e) Cognitive recovery is complete at 1 year

38 The adverse effects of benzodiazopines include:

(a) Confusion
(b) Aggression
(c) Cognitive deficits
(d) Respiratory depression
(e) Weight gain

37 (a) True
  (b) False
  (c) False
  (d) True
  (e) False

The time taken to regain continuous memory following the injury (post-traumatic amnesia or (PTA)) is a good predictor of prognosis:

(a) PTA <1 h   – return to work in 1 month;
(b) PTA <1 day   – return to work in 2 months;
(c) PTA <1 week   – return to work in 4 months.

Epilepsy is much less common following closed (5 per cent) than open (30 per cent) head injuries.

Post-concussional syndrome is relatively common (10–20 per cent in severe head injury).

Direct damage to the brain or the presence of bleeding worsen the prognosis.

Recovery of cognitive function following head trauma can be very slow and may continue over at least 2 years. The neuropsychological and neuropsychiatric consequences of even a relatively mild closed head injury include impairment of concentration and memory, as well as lability of mood, irritability and lack of energy.

38 (a) True
  (b) True
  (c) True
  (d) True
  (e) False

Benzodiazepines (e.g. Diazepam, Temazepam and Lorazepam) are extremely potent drugs which relieve anxiety rapidly and effectively *in the short term*. They do have a number of problems, not least that of dependence. Over-sedation and confusional states can occur, particularly in the elderly, in whom they are associated with falls. Some people have a paradoxical disinhibiting effect when taking Benzodiazepines, which can lead to violence. The reduction in vigilance induced by the drugs leads to problems with memory attention and problem solving. In overdose, especially when combined with alcohol, respiratory depression may cause death. At more therapeutic doses in those with a precarious respiratory drive, problems may ensue.

39 The following effects are mediated by the D_2 receptor activity of chlorpromazine:

   (a) Antipsychotic effect
   (b) Anti-emetic effect
   (c) Parkinsonian effect
   (d) Postural blood pressure drop
   (e) Weight gain

40 Tricyclic antidepressants:

   (a) Exert their effect by promoting monoamine reuptake
   (b) Can lower the seizure threshold
   (c) Can take up to 6 weeks to have a therapeutic effect
   (d) Diarrhoea is a common side-effect
   (e May precipitate mania

41 Bereavement:

   (a) Resolving a bereavement involves the person in reviewing episodes and feelings related to the bereavement
   (b) Is usually resolved in 3 months
   (c) Is not a cause of hallucinations
   (d) Counselling is always advisable after a bereavement
   (e) Counselling must be carried out by a psychiatrist

39 **(a) True**
 (b) True
 (c) False
 (d) False
 (e) False

Chlorpromazine (a potent antipsychotic medication) has effects on many receptors. The trade name Largactil derives from its large number of actions. The
antipsychotic effects are in part mediated via its occupancy of D_2 receptors, but it
is likely that the final story will be more complex than this. The anti-emetic effect
is mediated in this way. The development of Parkinsonian features works via D_1
receptors and postural hypotension via a blockade of alpha-1 noradrenaline
receptors. Weight gain is probably mediated via serotonin receptors.

When dealing with an acute psychiatric emergency, the use of intravenous
chlorpromazine is more hazardous than the use of intravenous haloperidol. First,
the phenothiazines have quinidine-like effects which are hazardous in patients
with pre-existing cardiac problems, whereas haloperidol does not carry this risk.
Second, phenothiazines are more likely to cause severe hypotension than
haloperidol. Chlorpromazine is more likely to cause seizures than haloperidol.

40 **(a) False**
 (b) True
 (c) True
 (d) False
 (e) True

Tricyclic antidepressants (e.g. Dothiepin, Amitriptyline) exert their action by
inhibiting the reuptake of amines (noradrenaline and serotonin (5HT)) into the
neurone. This potentiates their effect at the synapse. There is usually a delay
between starting the medication and the antidepressant response, and whilst this
is usually about 3 weeks, it may take up to 6 weeks before a response is seen.
Sedative and anxiolytic effects can develop within days. These drugs tend to lower
the seizure threshold and cause constipation rather than diarrhoea. They can
precipitate mania.

41 **(a) True**
 (b) False
 (c) False
 (d) False
 (e) False

Resolving the loss of a loved person through the different stages of mourning
(numbness, sadness and acceptance) happens by recalling events and feelings
related to the loss. This process is usually complete by about 6 months. Seeing
images of the dead person following a bereavement is such a common
phenomenon that it can be regarded as normal. Those experiencing it may
believe it is a symptom of mental illness. Counselling is indicated if there are
particular problems of delay, prolongation or intensity of these stages. There is no
particular value in psychiatrists carrying out this task, and most mental health
professionals have this skill. It has been demonstrated that, with training,
volunteers are able to carry out this work effectively.

42 In anorexia nervosa:

   (a) Sufferers have a distorted image of their body
   (b) Menstrual irregularities are more common than in bulimia nervosa
   (c) A body weight 25 per cent below that expected is required to make the diagnosis
   (d) Growth hormone levels are raised
   (e) Later age of onset is a poor prognostic sign

43 Opiate dependence leads to:

   (a) Constricted pupils
   (b) Hypersexuality
   (c) Diarrhoea
   (d) Shivering
   (e) Peripheral neuropathy
   (f) Psychosis

42 **(a) True**
   (b) True
   (c) False
   (d) True
   (e) True

Diagnostic criteria for anorexia nervosa:

(a) refusal to maintain a body weight that is at least 85 per cent of the minimum normal weight for the person's age, height and build;
(b) intense fear of gaining weight or becoming fat;
(c) a disturbance in the way in which the body is perceived;
(d) amenorrhoea.

As weight decreases in anorexia nervosa, body image disturbance increases. Severe medical complications of anorexia nervosa include very low systolic blood pressure, hypokalaemia and cardiac arrhythmias. In-patient treatment is indicated for those who develop these complications, or whose weight is 65 per cent below the mean matched population weight for height. Suicide risk is another indication for admission, as is rapid weight loss. In addition to raised growth hormone levels, there is an increase in plasma cortisol, with loss of normal circadian rhythm. Gonadotrophin levels are reduced. Hypokalaemia results from laxative abuse. In addition to anxiety about eating in public, the anorexic tends to want to cook for others, hides her weight loss with bulky clothes, and tends to deny being on a diet, or may claim to be a vegetarian.

43 **(a) True**
   (b) False
   (c) False
   (d) False
   (e) False
   (f) False

Opiate dependence can lead to constipation, suppression of the cough reflex and recurrent chest infections, as well as constricted pupils. The person's sex drive is usually reduced. Unlike the psychostimulants such as cocaine and amphetamines, opiate dependence does not cause hallucinations and delusions.

When examining a person who is suspected of abusing drugs, one should look for stigmata such as needle marks, skin abscesses and pupillary changes, and the signs of intoxication or withdrawal, as well as the presence of hepatitis B or C or HIV infection.

44 The Mental Health Act 1983:

   (a) Nurses can detain a patient for 72 h on Section 5 (4)
   (b) Section 2 requires only the recommendation of the person's GP
   (c) Section 4 requires only the recommendation of an approved social worker
   (d) ECT can be given only under the Mental Health Act
   (e) Psychosurgery can be performed only under the Mental Health Act

45 Delusions:

   (a) Are always accompanied by hallucinations
   (b) Are always false
   (c) Must be evaluated in the light of a person's cultural background
   (d) May be shared by two or more people
   (e) Become systematized in dementia

44 (a) **False**
   (b) **False**
   (c) **False**
   (d) **False**
   (e) **True**

The Mental Health Act 1983 (MHA) allows nursing staff to detain an already admitted person for up to 6 h on a section 5 (4) in order that they might be further assessed as soon as is practicable. Section 2 requires recommendations from either the person's GP and an approved psychiatrist (usually the consultant or specialist registrar) involved in the person's care, or two specially approved but independent doctors before an application is made by the social worker. Section 4 allows for emergency admission for 72 h by any doctor (usually the person's GP) in conjunction with an approved social worker, if there would be an unreasonable delay in getting assessment by two doctors. ECT may be given if informed consent for the treatment is given by its recipient. Psychosurgery can only be performed under the MHA following independent review.

45 (a) **False**
   (b) **False**
   (c) **True**
   (d) **True**
   (e) **False**

A delusion is a belief that is held with utter conviction despite evidence to the contrary, and that is not explicable by the educational, social or cultural background of the person. It is the result of pathological thought processes.

It is often the case that hallucinations and delusions go together, but it is not invariably so. Delusions may exist without hallucinations.

Beliefs must always be placed within the person's cultural background. In the multicultural society in which we live it is unlikely that we will all share common concepts of the world and the supernatural. A delusion may be shared by more than one person (*folie à deux*). Frequently a stronger partner draws a less robust one into the delusional system, which breaks down once the influence of the partner is removed.

In dementia, delusional ideas tend to be fragmentary and fleeting, unlike those in schizophrenia.

46 Obsessions:

    (a) Preoccupy the sufferer despite attempts to exclude them
    (b) Are felt to come from outside the person
    (c) The idea is generally known to be false
    (d) Resistance can diminish over time
    (e) Can occur in schizophrenia

47 Memory:

    (a) Memory loss for recent events is seen in Korsakov's syndrome
    (b) Retrograde amnesia is a good predictor of recovery from head injury.
    (c) Measures of memory function are stable in delirium.
    (d) Memory can be accurately assessed in the presence of a depressive illness.
    (e) Psychogenic amnesia has a slow onset

48 In mania:

    (a) Schneider's first-rank symptoms do not occur in mania
    (b) Insight is impaired
    (c) Sexual desires are decreased
    (d) Irritability is a common feature
    (e) Stupor is unknown

46 (a) True
   (b) False
   (c) True
   (d) True
   (e) True

Obsessions are recurrent, persistent thoughts, images or impulses which are experienced as intrusive and which cause anxiety and distress. They are not simply anxieties about real-life problems. The person attempts to resist them initially, but this resistance diminishes over time. They are recognized as being the product of the sufferer's own mind.

This symptom can occur in other disorders, most commonly in depression, but not infrequently in schizophrenia as well.

47 (a) True
   (b) False
   (c) False
   (d) False
   (e) False

In Korsakov's syndrome the person is unable to lay down any new memory, and will confabulate to cover the deficit.

Post-traumatic amnesia is a much better predictor of recovery from a head injury than the memory loss for the period prior to the injury (retrograde amnesia).

In delirium the mental state fluctuates widely, and this is reflected in tests of memory.

In depression the person has poor concentration and will often make little effort to engage in the testing. It may seem at first sight as if the person is suffering from a dementia (sometimes called a pseudodementia), but careful history-taking will reveal the presence of depressive symptoms before the memory problems emerged.

Psychogenic amnesia usually has an acute onset following an emotionally traumatic event.

48 (a) False
   (b) True
   (c) False
   (d) True
   (e) False

In mania, Schneider's first-rank symptoms occur in approximately 20 per cent of cases. The person has little insight into their mental state, and will become irritable with those who attempt to thwart their plans. Disinhibition can lead to an increase in sexual activity, which can have disastrous consequences as contraception and safe-sex practices are ignored. In extreme cases stupor can ensue, in which the person becomes ecstatic and completely out of touch with the world. During these periods they do not eat or drink, and need careful supportive management.

49 The following make a diagnosis of vascular dementia more likely than Alzheimer's disease:

(a) Smooth progression of the disease
(b) Hypertension
(c) Damage to the personality
(d) Neurological localizing signs
(e) Emotional lability

50 Factors associated with a good prognosis in schizophrenia are:

(a) Early age of onset
(b) A psychosocial precipitant to the episode
(c) Normal CT scan
(d) Gradual onset
(e) Positive symptoms

49 (a) **False**
   (b) **True**
   (c) **False**
   (d) **True**
   (e) **True**

Clinically it is often difficult to make a diagnosis of a specific dementia syndrome, but the following elements are usually considered:

Alzheimer's disease	Vascular dementia
Slow onset	Abrupt onset
Smooth progression	Stepwise progression
Normal blood pressure	Hypertension
No localizing neurological signs	Localizing neurological signs
No history of stroke	History of stroke
Personality change	Personality intact
Emotionally stable	Emotionally labile

Reduced survival is associated, in both Alzheimer's disease and vascular dementia, with the appearance of primitive reflexes such as a sucking reflex, snout reflex and glabellar tap reflex, which are indicative of a widespread diffuse cortical lesion.

50 (a) **False**
   (b) **True**
   (c) **True**
   (d) **False**
   (e) **True**

Table 2 Prognosis in schizophrenia

Good prognosis	Bad prognosis
Satisfactory social relationships, academic and work performance	Poor social relationships, academic and work performance
Later onset	Early onset
Rapid onset	Gradual onset
A psychosocial precipitant	No precipitant
Hallucinations and delusions (positive symptoms)	Paucity of thought, lack of activity, lack of affect (negative symptoms)
Normal CT scan	Abnormal CT scan
Good response to medication	Little response to medication

51 Deliberate self-harm:

(a) Has a higher incidence in inner cities
(b) 1–2 per cent of cases repeat the act within 1 year
(c) 10 per cent of cases will die of suicide during the next 2 years
(d) Repetition is predicted by higher social class
(e) Repetition is predicted by alcohol problems

51 (a) True
 (b) False
 (c) False
 (d) False
 (e) True

Following an act of deliberate self-harm careful assessment of the person's intent is important:

(a) presence or absence of a mental illness (15–25 per cent of cases have one);
(b) the perception by the individual of the seriousness of their act;
(c) was the attempt violent (e.g. hanging, shooting, leaping or drowning)?
(d) have they planned it?
(e) have they taken steps to avoid being found?
(f) was there a note?
(g) do they live alone?
(h) have they chronic ill health?
(j) was alcohol involved?

Deliberate self-harm is more common in urban environments, with repetition predicted by a lower social class and the presence of alcohol problems. Over the next year, 1–2 per cent will die by suicide (a risk 100 times higher than that of the general population). Twenty per cent will repeat the act within 1 year. Recently there has been an increase in completed suicides by young men, sometimes associated with unemployment, sometimes in association with schizophrenia.

Psychosocial problems that are commonly associated with deliberate self-harm include marital and family disharmony, problems at work, study difficulties, debt, poor housing and harassment by neighbours, prosecution, conviction or imprisonment, substance abuse, severe physical illness and social isolation (Bancroft, J., Skrimshire, A., Casson, J. *et al.* 1977: People who deliberately poison or injure themselves: their problems and their contacts with helping agencies. *Psychological Medicine* **7**, 289–303).

52 Dementia may be caused by:

  (a) Systemic lupus erythematosus
  (b) HIV infection
  (c) Hypothyroidism
  (d) Syphilis
  (e) Rheumatoid disease

52 **(a) True**
   (b) True
   (c) True
   (d) True
   (e) False

A list of the causes of dementing illnesses would probably fill this book and several more besides! Vascular dementia, Alzheimer's disease and, increasingly recognized, Lewy body dementia are the three most common types of dementia. Other causes or 'treatable' causes are rare but must not be missed. The standard 'Dementia Screen' consists of careful history taking from an informant, physical examination and blood tests, supplemented with imaging and EEG studies where the level of suspicion is high.

Routine laboratory tests in dementia (Dementia Screen) include the following:
(a) full blood count (FBC);
(b) erythrocyte sedimentation rate (ESR);
(c) urea and electrolytes (U&Es);
(d) liver function tests (LFTs);
(e) calcium and phosphate (Ca^{++} and PO_4^{--});
(f) syphilis serology;
(g) vitamin B_{12} and folate;
(h) blood sugar;
(i) urine culture.

Having rheumatoid arthritis seems to protect against developing dementia, perhaps as a result of non-steroidal anti-inflammatory medication.

53 The following are true of post-traumatic stress disorder (PTSD):

   (a) Persistent hypoarousal
   (b) Sleep disturbance
   (c) Flashbacks ('action replay' of the traumatic incident)
   (d) Good response to medication
   (e) Seeking reminders of the trauma

54 Foods and drinks to avoid with monoamine oxidase inhibitors (MAOIs) include:

   (a) Bananas
   (b) Fortified wine
   (c) Low-alcohol lager
   (d) Camembert cheese
   (e) Pickled herrings

53 **(a) False**
　(b) True
　(c) True
　(d) False
　(e) False

The diagnostic features of post-traumatic stress disorder are:

(a) exposure to an event which threatens death or serious injury of themselves or others;
(b) the response to this being intense fear and helplessness;
(c) persistent avoidance of stimuli that remind the person of the event;
(d) persistent symptoms of increased arousal, e.g. sleep disturbance, outbursts of anger, poor concentration;
(e) the events being re-experienced e.g. in flashbacks or dreams.

The disorder is more likely to occur after 'man-made' events than after natural disasters. It responds poorly to medication.

Survivor guilt is a term used to describe an irrational sense that the survivor's life was 'purchased at the cost of another's'. Sources of survivor guilt derive from relief at not having died oneself, guilt for failing to save the victim (however irrational this might be), guilt about those who might have died as a result of one's own actions (again however irrational that might be), and guilt over being 'undeserving of having been saved' (Raphael, B. 1986: *When disaster strikes.* London: Hutchinson).

54 **(a) False**
　(b) True
　(c) True
　(d) True
　(e) True

The classical monoamine oxidase inhibitors (e.g. Phenelzine, Tranylcypramine) bind irreversibly to the enzyme and are unselective about the form to which they bind (A or B). In so doing, they block the activity of the enzyme in the gut wall, allowing the passage of tyramine into the blood. The tyramine is converted into noradrenaline and released both centrally and peripherally, causing a hypertensive crisis. The following tyramine-rich foods must be avoided:

(a) cheese;
(b) pickled herring;
(c) broad bean pods;
(d) Bovril, Oxo, Marmite;
(e) alcoholic drinks (even with low alcohol content);
(f) game.

There is now available a reversible inhibitor of monoamine oxidase A (RIMA) called moclobemide (Manerix) which is much safer than the irreversible forms.

55 The side-effects of tricyclic antidepressants include:

   (a) Urinary retention
   (b) Clubbing
   (c) Convulsions
   (d) Anorgasmia
   (e) Dysmenorrhoea

56 Acute symptoms of benzodiazepine withdrawal include:

   (a) Stupor
   (b) Convulsions
   (c) Hallucinations
   (d) Rebound insomnia
   (e) Ataxia

55 **(a) True**
   (b) False
   (c) True
   (d) True
   (e) False

Tricyclic antidepressants are highly effective in treating depression but have a number of side-effects which limit their usefulness.

Anti-cholinergic: urinary retention, dry mouth, constipation, confusion, blurred vision, glaucoma, cardiac dysrhythmias and sexual dysfunction.

Anti-adrenergic: sedation and postural hypotension.

Quinidine-like: cardiac dysrythmias, reduction of the fit threshold and excess sweating.

56 **(a) False**
   (b) True
   (c) True
   (d) True
   (e) True

The problem of dependence upon benzodiazepines is a common one, and the symptoms experienced on withdrawal are as follows.

Psychological symptoms:

  (a) anxiety;
  (b) apprehension;
  (c) insomnia;
  (d) dysphoria;
  (e) in extreme cases, confusional states and paranoia;
  (f) hallucinations.

Somatic symptoms:

  (a) palpitations;
  (b) tremor;
  (c) vertigo;
  (d) sweating;
  (e) hypersensitivity to light, noise and pain;
  (f) ataxia;
  (g) convulsions.

57 Selective serotonin reuptake inhibitors (SSRIs):

    (a) Are safer in overdose than tricyclic antidepressants
    (b) Increase the convulsion threshold
    (c) Have a high incidence of gastrointestinal side-effects
    (d) May interfere with the metabolism of warfarin
    (e) Can be effective in obsessive-compulsive disorder

58 Akathisia is characterized by the following:

    (a) A sense of internal restlessness
    (b) Partially relieved by pacing
    (c) Caused by chronic benzodiazepine abuse
    (d) Not caused by clozapine
    (e) Alleviated by beta blockers

57 (a) True
   (b) False
   (c) True
   (d) True
   (e) True

The introduction of the SSRIs was a significant step forward in the management of depressive illnesses. They are much less toxic than the tricyclic antidepressants whose cardiac effects are so dangerous in overdose. Like the tricyclic antidepressants, they reduce the convulsion threshold and must be used with care in those with epilepsy. Their main side-effects are gastrointestinal. These usually abate in time, but are a common reason for stopping the drug. They can interfere with the metabolism of warfarin, leading to bleeding. The SSRIs can be effective in obsessive-compulsive disorder, usually at higher doses than in depression.

58 (a) True
   (b) True
   (c) False
   (d) True
   (e) True

This is a drug-induced extrapyramidal syndrome consisting of an intense and uncomfortable sense of inner restlessness associated with pacing and stereo-typed restless movements. It is partially relieved by walking around, and is made worse when the person lies down or sits still. Akathisia contributes to a refusal to take medication, and is so distressing that it can result in suicide. Akathisia might be relieved by a reduction in the dose of neuroleptic or switching to risperidone or clozapine. Propranolol, clonidine, antihistimine and benzodiazepines can also be used for this distressing condition. It can occur in between 25 and 50 per cent of people treated with neuroleptics (Barnes, T. R. E. 1987: The present status of tardive dyskinesia and akathisia in the treatment of schizophrenia. *Psychiatric Developments* **4**, 301–29).

59 A psychogenic cause for male impotence is suggested by:

    (a) A recent stressful life event
    (b) Loss of erections on waking
    (c) Previous uninterrupted normal sexual functioning
    (d) An inability to masturbate
    (e) Problems in the relationship

60 The following are characteristic of opiate withdrawal:

    (a) Sleepiness
    (b) Lacrimation
    (c) Abdominal pain
    (d) Constricted pupils
    (e) Yawning

59 (a) True
   (b) False
   (c) False
   (d) False
   (e) True

It is often the case that one cannot identify a purely organic or purely psychogenic cause for impotence, and that the two interact. However, a number of features give some clues.

Table 3 Organic and psychogenic causes

Organic causes	Psychogenic causes
No recent life event	Recent life event
With all partners	With only one partner
Inability to masturbate	Ability to masturbate
Loss of erections on waking	Erections on waking
No relationship problems prior to the impotence	Relationship problems prior to the impotence
Abnormalities on physical examination	Normal physical examination

60 (a) False
   (b) True
   (c) True
   (d) False
   (e) True

The symptoms of opiate withdrawal are:

(a) lack of sleep;
(b) lacrimation;
(c) abdominal pain, often with diarrhoea;
(d) dilated pupils;
(e) yawning;
(f) gooseflesh;
(g) shivering;
(h) restlessness;
(i) muscle pain;
(j) sweating.

The symptoms may be alleviated with controlled withdrawal using methadone.

61 The following is true of depression in the elderly:

    (a) At 1 year only one in three is fully recovered
    (b) Initial prognosis is good, but relapse is high
    (c) Prognosis is poorer in the lower social classes
    (d) ECT is contraindicated
    (e) Nihilistic delusions may be present

62 A pathological grief reaction is suggested by:

    (a) The development of behaviour resembling that of the dead person
    (b) Searching behaviour in the first 3 weeks
    (c) Intense grief between 3 and 6 weeks
    (d) Intense anger and depression after 6 months
    (e) The first signs of grieving after an interval of more than 2 months

61 (a) True
   (b) True
   (c) True
   (d) False
   (e) True

The treatment of depression in the elderly is often very satisfying, with a fairly rapid return to normal functioning. However, in uncontrolled studies to date there has been a high rate of relapse in the first year, and often residual symptoms are noted. The outcome is worse in the lower social classes. One reason for this state of affairs is perhaps that treatment has not been as vigorous as in younger people, nor has it gone on for as long as it should have done. Whilst the rates of complication for ECT in the elderly are higher than in younger people (especially confusional states), it is a highly effective treatment even in the very frail and those who suffer from both dementia and depression.

Nihilistic delusions (e.g. I am dead, I am rotting) can be present and are known as Cotard's syndrome.

62 (a) True
   (b) False
   (c) False
   (d) True
   (e) True

The 'stunned' phase, in which the emotions are blunted, typically lasts for between a few hours to 2 weeks at the most. The next phase is one of fear, distress, sleeplessness and loss of appetite. The bereaved individual might talk incoherently about their loss. In general people do not mimic the behaviour of the dead person (identification), but may well respond as if they were there still for some time – e.g. looking around when there are noises in the house, inadvertently setting two places at the table – or experience symptoms resembling the dead person's illness. The stages may be prolonged or delayed, which postpones the person getting back to a reasonably normal state.

The mourning phase is one of preoccupation with the deceased. There may be denial, guilt and/or transient hallucinatory episodes. Anger, directed at fate, medical staff or aimed at oneself for allowing the death to occur is a common feature at this stage, as are guilt, denial and transient hallucinatory experiences. There are feelings of intense unhappiness and despair with tearfulness, sighing, intense yearning and distress. Within several weeks after the loss, the bereaved progresses to the phase of acceptance and adjustment. Atypical grief is described by Murray Parkes as a protracted bereavement reaction lasting for well over 6 months and characterized by ideas of worthlessness, guilt, denial and failure to resume normal household or professional activities. The bereaved person might present to a GP with 'functional' pain which is located at the site of the deceased's terminal illness, e.g. abdominal pain in the case of a spouse who has died of carcinoma of the stomach.

63 Learning disabilities:

- (a) Are more common in females than in males
- (b) There is an additional X chromosome in people with Klinefelter's syndrome
- (c) Single-gene abnormalities are rare
- (d) Phenylketonuria is the commonest single recessive gene abnormality
- (e) Babies with phenylketonuria appear abnormal from birth

64 Down's syndrome
- (a) Is the commonest cause of severe learning difficulty
- (b) The risk is diminished with maternal age
- (c) About 50 per cent of the sufferers develop an Alzheimer-like dementia by the age of 50 years
- (d) The diagnosis can be predicted by sampling maternal cerebrol-spinal fluid
- (e) Heart abnormalities are rare

63 **(a) False**
   (b) True
   (c) True
   (d) True
   (e) False

The main causes of learning disability include Down's syndrome (26 per cent), perinatal injury (18 per cent), unknown (15 per cent), post-infective (14 per cent), other inherited conditions (10 per cent), congenital abnormalities (9 per cent) and metabolic causes (4 per cent). It should be noted that these proportions vary depending upon the severity of the impairment, e.g. genetic causes are much more common in those with severe compared to mild learning disability. Life expectancy has increased during this century, partly due to improved living conditions (as with the population in general) and partly due to specific intervention, such as cardiac surgery in Down's syndrome. People with learning disabilities have an increased morbidity with regard to the cardiovascular and respiratory systems, as well as orthopaedic problems, epilepsy and hearing and sight problems.

Learning disability is more common in males than in females by about 15 per cent in the community. Klinefelter's syndrome has the sex chromosomes XXY.

A very large number of single-gene abnormalities can cause learning disabilities, but each one is very rare. Of these, phenylketonuria is the commonest recessive gene abnormality, with an incidence of 12/1 000 000. Babies with phenylketonuria are normal at birth, but develop problems at about 3 months of age. Screening is with a simple blood test obtained by heel prick, and treatment is by diet.

64 **(a) True**
   (b) False
   (c) True
   (d) False
   (e) False

Down's syndrome (Trisomy 21) occurs in about 100/100 000 live births, with a further 15/100 000 pregnancies terminated as a result of screening. The risk of giving birth to a baby with Down's syndrome increases with the mother's age, but can be predicted from blood sampling (alpha-fetoprotein, unconjugated oestriol and human chorionic growth hormone). Ultrasound scanning is becoming increasingly sophisticated in its ability to identify fetuses with Down's syndrome, but sampling of fetal cells by amniocentesis confirms the diagnosis. Down's syndrome is associated with cardiac and gastrointestinal abnormalities and an increased incidence of leukaemia. About 55 per cent of sufferers from Down's syndrome develop dementia by the age of 50, the changes in the brain being like those of Alzheimer's disease. A wide range of physical abnormalities are found in the heart, gut, eyes, skin and teeth.

65 Psychiatric illness and learning disability:

   (a) Psychiatric illness is no more common in those with learning disability than in the general population

   (b) The presentation of psychiatric illness in learning disability is no different to that in the general population

   (c) Antidepressants need to be given in the same doses as for other depressed people

   (d) Antipsychotics need to be given in the same doses as for others in the population for whom they are prescribed

   (e) Schizophrenia has the same prognosis in those with and without learning disabilities

66 Child psychiatric disorders:

   (a) Are more common in rural areas

   (b) Conduct disorder is equally common in girls and boys

   (c) Speech and language delay predict later psychiatric disorder

   (d) Chronic physical illness is associated with a higher morbidity rate

   (e) Epilepsy does not increase the likelihood of psychiatric disorder in children

67 Conduct disorder:

   (a) The peak incidence is in the under-sevens

   (b) Is usually referred to psychiatric services soon after its inception

   (c) Boys are afflicted as often as girls

   (d) Depression and anxiety are commonly present

   (e) Is synonymous with delinquency

65 (a) **False**
   (b) **False**
   (c) **True**
   (d) **False**
   (e) **False**

Psychiatric illness is significantly more common in those who experience learning disabilities. The presentation of these illnesses is very different as the sufferers do not have the same language skills, coping abilities or impulse control. When a person with learning difficulties requires an antidepressant, they usually require it in the same dose as others who are depressed. Care must be taken not to induce epilepsy, as this group of people is very sensitive to the side-effects. This is even more marked when antipsychotic medications are used, and they are frequently required in lower than average doses. Schizophrenia in a person with learning difficulties has a poor prognosis.

66 (a) **False**
   (b) **False**
   (c) **True**
   (d) **True**
   (e) **False**

As with most psychiatric disorders, child psychiatric disorders have a higher prevalence in cities. Conduct disorder is the commonest childhood disorder, but it is more often associated with boys than girls, whilst emotional disorders are equally distributed until adolescence, when they become more common in females. Speech and language delay at 3 years old is significantly associated with later disorders. Chronic physical illnesses and epilepsy are associated with an increase in the rate of psychiatric disorders. For those with active epilepsy, the rate is 35 per cent.

67 (a) **False**
   (b) **False**
   (c) **False**
   (d) **True**
   (e) **False**

Conduct disorder is characterized by behavioural disturbance (aggression, stealing, lying and destructiveness). It is the commonest psychiatric disorder of older children and teenagers, rather than the under-sevens. It is three times more common in boys than in girls. It has usually been present for some considerable time before the family are referred to services. Often associated with family morbidity, children with conduct disorder often have symptoms of anxiety and depression.

Delinquency is a legal term referring to breaking the law in the under–17s. Many delinquents are not psychiatrically disordered.

68 Depressive illness in childhood:

    (a) Is more common in girls pre-pubertally
    (b) Is more common in boys post-pubertally
    (c) Post-pubertally is associated with a family history of depression
    (d) May be a cause of school refusal
    (e) Is not a cause of antisocial behaviour

69 Hyperkinetic syndrome:

    (a) Different definitions of the disorder have led to a 20-fold difference in prevalence rates
    (b) Using strict criteria (ICD-9) the prevalence rate is 5 per cent
    (c) The incidence is the same in both sexes
    (d) Over time the hyperkinesis declines
    (e) Amphetamines are contraindicated

70 Autism:

    (a) Children with autism have abnormalities of language development
    (b) Non-verbal communication is unaffected
    (c) Autistic children welcome change and novelty
    (d) Is a single homogenous disorder
    (e) Autistic children find abstract thought difficult

68 **(a) False**
   (b) False
   (c) True
   (d) True
   (e) False

In pre-pubertal children, depressive illnesses are more common in boys than in girls and are associated with family problems such as alcoholism and antisocial behaviour. Post-pubertally girls outnumber boys, and the illness is more likely to be primary and associated with a family history of depressive illness. Both school refusal and antisocial behaviour may be a consequence of depressive illnesses.

69 **(a) True**
   (b) False
   (c) False
   (d) True
   (e) False

The concept of hyperkinetic syndrome has been controversial, with huge variations between the USA and UK definitions of the disorder. This has led to prevalence rates in different studies varying 20 fold. When strict ICD-9 criteria are applied, the prevalence rate is 0.1 per cent. The onset is usually before 3 years, with boys affected three times more often than girls. There is often a history of neurodevelopmental abnormalities, distractibility and poor attention span. Over time the hyperkinesis diminishes, but the attention problems remain, leading to poor school performance.

Paradoxically, amphetamines (Pemoline and methylphenidate) reduce the child's activity levels, improving the quality of interactions that the child has with others, but doing little to improve their academic performance.

70 **(a) True**
   (b) False
   (c) False
   (d) False
   (e) True

Autism is a rare condition (affecting 4.5/10 000 children). There are abnormalities of cognition, socialization, language development and abnormal behaviour with little development of non-verbal communication. The behaviour of autistic children is rigid and stereotyped. They also experience a wide range of non-specific behavioural abnormalities, such as overactivity, tantrums and head-banging.

It is unlikely to be a homogenous disorder with both genes and brain damage implicated in its development. Half of the cases of autism are associated with specific abnormalities such as tuberose sclerosis or phenylketonuria.

Some children become very skilled at mechanical or repetitive tasks, but lack abstract or imaginative thought.

71 Sleep disorders:

   (a) Insomnia is defined as less than 6 h of sleep a night
   (b) Most disorders of sleep are secondary
   (c) People with Kleine-Levin syndrome suffer from decreased sleep
   (d) Narcolepsy is associated with HLA DR2
   (e) Exercise late at night is conducive to sleep

72 General practice:

   (a) Only 70 per cent of people are registered with a general practitioner
   (b) General practitioners report similar rates of mental illness from one practice to another
   (c) Mental illness represents 20 per cent of general practice consultations
   (d) Most mental health consultations will be for psychotic illnesses
   (e) Questionnaire studies underestimate the level of psychiatric morbidity in general practice

71 **(a) False**
   (b) True
   (c) False
   (d) True
   (e) False

Insomnia is essentially a subjective phenomenon, with the affected person reporting that they have poor quantity or quality of sleep regardless of the time actually spent asleep. Most sleep disorders are secondary. A careful history excluding psychiatric disorder, physical causes, e.g. pain or prostate problems, or drugs, e.g. caffeine, must be taken.

People who suffer from Kleine-Levin syndrome suffer from *excess* sleep lasting days or weeks, accompanied by intense hunger. Narcolepsy is associated with HLA DR2.

Sleep hygienists recommend a careful routine before retiring to sleep. This includes reducing tea, coffee, alcohol and other fluid intake, sleeping where it is warm and comfortable, eating only light snacks in the evening, and confining exercise to the late afternoon or early evening.

72 **(a) False**
   (b) False
   (c) True
   (d) False
   (e) False

One of the great strengths of general practice in the UK is that 98 per cent of the population are registered with a GP; 70 per cent of people and 90 per cent of families will see their GP in any year. GPs vary enormously (9-fold) in their estimates of mental illness within their practices, despite the fact that 20 per cent of their consultations pertain to mental illness. This variation depends on the GP's ability to recognize mental illness, which frequently presents in a covert manner with physical problems. Psychotic illnesses such as schizophrenia and bipolar affective disorder are relatively rare in general practice. Most problems are of a 'neurotic' nature, with admixtures of depression and anxiety.

Questionnaire surveys of general practice attendees tend to *overestimate* the levels of psychiatric illness, producing many false positives.

73 Detection of psychiatric disorder in general practice:

    (a) Is unlikely if the person has both physical and mental disorders
    (b) Is not influenced by people's expectations of the doctor
    (c) Is more likely if information is given by the doctor early in the consultation
    (d) Makes no difference to subsequent consultation rates
    (e) Has an impact on physical problems

74 Epilepsy:

    (a) Psychotic symptoms are unlikely as part of an aura
    (b) The suicide rate of those with epilepsy is the same as that of the general population
    (c) Pseudo-seizures and epilepsy can coexist in the same person
    (d) Age of onset of epilepsy is not associated with cognitive impairment
    (e) Schizophrenia-like episodes without EEG abnormalities occur in those with epilepsy

73 **(a) True**
   (b) False
   (c) False
   (d) False
   (e) True

Detection of psychiatric disorder in general practice depends on factors related both to the GP and also to the person consulting them. Many people use a physical problem as an entrée into the GP's surgery, as they expect that this will interest their doctor, feeling that doctors do not deal with psychological problems. People who present with physical problems are less likely to have their mental health problems recognized If there is also a clearly organic problem present as well as a mental health problem, then the likelihood of detection is even lower.

   GPs who make good eye contact, interrupt less and give information *only at the end of the consultation* are more likely to detect mental health problems than their colleagues. Detection of mental health problems leads to a reduction in the consultation rate of the sufferers, and also to an improvement in any physical symptoms from which they suffer.

74 **(a) False**
   (b) False
   (c) True
   (d) False
   (e) True

Psychotic symptoms (delusions and hallucinations) can occur:

   (a) As part of the aura of epilepsy;
   (b) As part of the seizure itself (with impaired consciousness);
   (c) As a post-ictal phenomenon (usually with impaired consciousness);
   (d) Between seizures with EEG abnormalities not amounting to seizure (with impaired consciousness);
   (e) Between seizures, with a normal EEG (with consciousness not impaired).

Pseudo-seizures are often seen in those with 'true' epilepsy. A normal EEG during the 'fit' is diagnostic, but other clinical features may help to distinguish between the two.

Pseudo-seizures :

   (a) follow a psychological trauma;
   (b) have no aura;
   (c) are not associated with a fall, tongue-biting or incontinence;
   (d) have purposeful movements without the involvement of the abdominal muscles;
   (e) have no post-ictal effects;
   (f) blood prolactin is raised after true but not after pseudo-seizures.

75 HIV infection:

    (a) Mental disturbances occur at sero-conversion
    (b) Psychiatric problems only occur in response to learning of the infection, and at times of progression
    (c) Cognitive impairment occurs when the CD4 count is below 400
    (d) *Toxoplasma gondii* infection can cause changes in mental functioning
    (e) The presence of HIV in the brain causes 'functional' psychiatric illnesses

76 Psychiatry and childbirth:

    (a) Most disturbances of mood following childbirth resolve rapidly
    (b) One in every 500 births is accompanied by psychotic breakdown
    (c) Electroconvulsive therapy (ECT) is contraindicated following childbirth
    (d) An episode of puerperal depression does not increase the likelihood of a further episode in later life
    (e) Chronic depression postpartum is associated with an instrumental delivery

75 **(a) False**
   (b) False
   (c) True
   (d) True
   (e) True

Sero-conversion causes a flu-like illness with a general malaise. Rarely it can cause an encephalitis. Psychiatric problems are the result not only of the devastating news of infection and at times of disease progression (making pre- and post-test counselling and continuing support vital), but also of direct infection of the brain by the virus (mimicking all of the functional psychiatric disorders), secondary infections (e.g. *Toxoplasma gondii*) and mass lesions (e.g. lymphomas). Any change in the mental state of a person known to be HIV-positive demands careful neurological examination and appropriate neuro-imaging. Cognitive impairment is very rare unless there is evidence of immunosuppression (e.g. a CD4 count of <400).

In a person known to be HIV-positive who develops an acute organic state (delirium) with fluctuations in attention, concentration, memory and perception with emotional lability, it is important to detect the underlying cause, which might include:

  (a)   CNS opportunistic infections;
  (b)   intracranial space-occupying lesions;
  (c)   septicaemia;
  (d)   electrolyte imbalance;
  (e)   hypoxia;
  (f)   cerebral oedema;
  (g)   drug side-effects.

76 **(a) True**
   (b) True
   (c) False
   (d) False
   (e) False

Three types of disturbance are commonly seen following childbirth. Maternity blues is the commonest, affecting 50–70 per cent of women. It usually starts on the third or fourth day, and resolves over a couple more days. No specific treatment beyond support and reassurance is required.

Psychotic illnesses occur at a rate of one per 500 births. Most are affective in nature, about 20 per cent having features of schizophrenia. The mothers and their babies need specialist treatment to ensure the safety of both. ECT is a highly effective treatment for mothers who suffer in this way, and is *not* contraindicated.

Ten to 15 per cent of mothers develop depression within a few weeks of the child's birth; 5 per cent develop more chronic illnesses. These are usually associated with adverse life events, stress in the family, a history of depression and lack of social support, rather than complications of the delivery. Support from community midwives and health visitors is vital for this vulnerable group, who find it difficult to adjust to their new routines.

77 Psychotropic drugs and pregnancy/childbirth:

    (a) Lithium is safe in pregnancy
    (b) Lithium is secreted in the breast milk
    (c) Selective serotonin reuptake inhibitors (SSRIs) do not cross the placenta
    (d) Opiate withdrawal may precipitate premature labour
    (e) Withdrawal symptoms begin immediately after birth in the child of an opiate addict maintained on methadone

78 Anthropology and psychiatry:

    (a) Social causes of illness are regarded as more important in western industrialized societies
    (b) Immigrants have a higher rate of mental illness than their fellow country-men who stay at home
    (c) Distress is expressed in similar ways amongst all cultures
    (d) Purposeless self-injury is a part of the universal stereotype of madness
    (e) Belief in witchcraft can only act as a precipitant of mental disorder

77 (a) False
  (b) True
  (c) False
  (d) True
  (e) False

Lithium is contraindicated in pregnancy. It is associated with abnormalities in the fetus such as cleft palate and cardiac abnormalities. All women of reproductive age must be offered appropriate contraceptive advice when on lithium and advised about the balance of risk of fetal damage and relapse if they choose to start a family.

Lithium is secreted in the breast milk and can become toxic to the child, particularly if they develop diarrhoea.

Selective serotonin reuptake inhibitors (SSRIs) do cross the placenta. It is not clear that they cause any harm to the fetus but the manufacturers advise caution.

Opiate withdrawal may cause premature labour, fetal distress and even the death of the fetus. Ideally, withdrawal should take place in a slow, controlled manner at least 2 months before the baby is due. If this is not possible, then maintaining the mother on the lowest possible dose of methadone is advised. Following delivery by a mother maintained on methadone, the baby may not show any withdrawal signs for 48 or even 72 h. The baby must therefore be monitored very carefully.

78 (a) False
  (b) True
  (c) False
  (d) True
  (e) False

Arthur Kleinman developed the idea of Explanatory Models to include the culture-specific ideas that a person brings to explain their illness, as well as the individual's unique contribution. In western societies, environmental and physiological causes are deemed to be more important than in non-industrialized societies, where social or supernatural causes may be invoked.

Immigrants generally have a higher level of mental illness than either the population from which they originate or that to which they gravitate. This may be because they are a self-selected group at the margins of society, or it may be that migration itself induces stress.

Idioms of distress vary widely from culture to culture. In many societies psychological distress is expressed in bodily terms, particularly where the western notion of the mind-body split is not adopted. However, there are some behaviours which are universally recognized as 'mad', namely unprovoked violence, incomprehensible speech, gross self-neglect and purposeless self-injury. A belief in witchcraft may be a precipitant of mental disorder, or a part of the content of mental disorder, or the reason why someone believes that they are suffering from a mental disorder.

79 Fatigue:

- (a) 30 per cent of primary care attenders report fatigue as a symptom
- (b) Chronic fatigue syndrome is the only medical disorder to exist by Act of Parliament
- (c) Chronic fatigue syndrome has a better outcome if there is a coexistent psychiatric disorder
- (d) A belief in the 'physical' nature of their fatigue leads to a better outcome for sufferers of chronic fatigue syndrome
- (e) It is rare for fatigue to be iatrogenic

80 Borderline personality disorder:

- (a) The border is with affective disorders
- (b) There is a genetic component in its aetiology
- (c) The majority of cases are male
- (d) Self-mutilation is common
- (e) 10 per cent die by suicide

79 (a) False
   (b) True
   (c) True
   (d) False
   (e) False

Fatigue is a complaint reported by of about 10 per cent of general practice attenders. Tired all the time (TATT) attenders at the surgery are often difficult to deal with in a limited time and their problems are multi-factorial.

Much debate has surrounded the concept of chronic fatigue syndrome (CFS). As some authorities did not recognize its existence, sufferers had a difficult time receiving appropriate sickness benefits. Eventually, Parliament passed a statute recognizing the illness as one that was deserving of the same consideration as any other illness. If the person with CFS presents with overt psychiatric symptoms such as anxiety and depression which can be managed in their own right, the outlook for them is brighter than for those who are entrenched in the view that their problems have no psychological basis and that they will become well when the correct physical treatment for their as yet undiscovered pathogen is given.

It is not unusual for doctors to be the cause of fatigue; Many commonly prescribed drugs cause fatigue. Many psychotropic drugs produce fatigue as a side-effect, but drugs such as diuretics and beta blockers should not be forgotten either.

80 (a) False
   (b) True
   (c) False
   (d) True
   (e) True

Borderline personality disorder is one of the commonest personality disorders. Those who suffer from it live in intense fear of rejection and loss. They are very sensitive to environmental cues, and change rapidly in their mental state. The changes include brief psychotic episodes (borderline with psychosis). Seventy-five per cent of those suffering are women. Borderline personality disorder is five times more common in the first-degree relatives of sufferers than in the general population. In circumstances of acute distress the sufferers will often mutilate themselves, which brings them into contact with the psychiatric services; 10 per cent go on to complete their suicide.

81 Alcohol:

   (a) Those with Korsakoff's Syndrome are aware of their memory deficits
   (b) Alcohol withdrawal fits may occur up to 1 month after withdrawal
   (c) The mamillary bodies are damaged in Korsakoff's syndrome
   (d) Total abstinence is the treatment goal for all with problem drinking
   (e) Chlormethiazole (Hemineverin) is the drug of choice in alcohol withdrawal

82 Assessment of the drug abuser:

   (a) The reason for presentation at this time does not matter
   (b) What they say that they are taking is important
   (c) Physical examination adds little to the assessment
   (d) The amount of money spent on drugs is the most reliable indicator of use
   (e) Prescription drugs need not be considered

81 (a) **False**
　　(b) **False**
　　(c) **True**
　　(d) **False**
　　(e) **False**

Those who suffer from Korsakoff's Syndrome have little insight into their inability to learn new material and confabulate to cover up the deficits. In both Wernicke's encephalopathy and Korsakoff's syndrome there is haemorrhage into the mamillary bodies and the medial dorsal nuclei of the thalamus.

Withdrawal fits may take place up to 2 weeks following the cessation of drinking.

Total abstinence is probably the ideal state for those who have experienced problem drinking but for those under 40 years of age and who have sustained no physical damage, controlled drinking may be a reasonable goal.

Chlormethiazole (Hemineverin) has a long and creditable history for alcohol detoxification. It is highly addictive and can be difficult to withdraw. If taken with alcohol it may cause death and its use as an intravenous infusion for those in delirium tremens, where it was particularly dangerous, has been superseded Benzodiazepines can be used (e.g. Diazepam), and although some of the same problems apply, these drugs are by and large safer and their effects can be reversed. Carbemazepine is many peoples' first-line drug as it avoids many of the dependency effects of the other drugs. Any withdrawal regime should be accompanied by 300 mg tds of thiamine to protect against Wernicke's encephalopathy and Korsakoff's syndrome.

82 (a) **False**
　　(b) **True**
　　(c) **False**
　　(d) **True**
　　(e) **False**

Drug abusers come in all shapes and sizes. Few conform to the media stereotypes, so a detailed assessment of each is important. The motivation for presentation will vary widely and should be looked at carefully, as it will influence the type of intervention proposed and the likely outcome of that intervention. Whilst the history of drug use may be unreliable, many drug abusers are stable in their usage and can give details of this. It should be noted that street drugs vary enormously in their potency and quality from batch to batch. The amount of money spent on the drugs may give a clearer idea of how much is being used, if you are aware of the going rate. Physical examination is important. Look for signs of intoxication or withdrawal, puncture marks, scars or abscesses which suggest intravenous use and hence an increased risk of HIV infection, cardiovascular state (listen for the murmurs of SBE) and the jaundice of hepatitis B.

Many drug abusers abuse prescription drugs, particularly analgesics and benzodiazepines. All practices are familiar with the person presenting to different doctors demanding fresh supplies of drugs before their prescription should have run out.

83 Solvent abuse:

    (a) Usually takes place alone
    (b) Is commoner among boys
    (c) Ten per cent experience visual hallucinations
    (d) Causes physical dependency
    (e) Causes death by brain damage

84 When interviewing a person with mental health problems:

    (a) Your non-verbal communication is unimportant
    (b) The arrangement of the furniture is important
    (c) It is important to describe the person's problems in medical language
    (d) Sharing your understanding of the person is undesirable
    (e) It is unlikely that the person will remember much of what you have said

83 (a) **False**
   (b) **True**
   (c) **False**
   (d) **False**
   (e) **False**

Solvent abuse is usually a communal activity undertaken by boys between the ages of 8 and 19 years. The effects of euphoria, disorientation, blurred vision, ataxia and nausea usually last about 2 h, and 40 per cent of solvent abusers experience visual hallucinations. There is no withdrawal syndrome or physical dependency. Death is caused by cardiac dysrhythmias (particularly at times of physical exertion), respiratory depression, asphyxia, inhalation of vomit and trauma, but not by direct brain damage.

84 (a) **False**
   (b) **True**
   (c) **False**
   (d) **False**
   (e) **True**

When talking to a person with mental health problems (or anyone else for that matter) your non-verbal behaviour is of vital importance. Sitting in an attentive pose, nodding and encouraging will create an atmosphere that promotes disclosure. The arrangement of the furniture is also very important. It is difficult to interview across a large expanse of desk. It is much better to get a verbatim account of the person's problems. Get them to expand on terms such as 'depression' which have both a lay and a medical usage – they may not mean what you mean. It will also help when sharing your understanding of their problem if you are able to provide feedback in words that the person uses, rather than unintelligible medicalese. As people take away very little of what is said to them during medical consultations, using their own language will help them to remember. Repetition and recapitulation helps you both to clarify where you are. Writing things down for the person to take away can be very useful.

85 A Mental State:

    (a) This is done separately to the history taking
    (b) Describes the person's psychopathology only at the time of interview
    (c) It is important to include biological features of depression under mood
    (d) You can assume that a person is experiencing hallucinations from their behaviour
    (e) Should include a description of your surroundings

86 Violent behaviour:

    (a) There is greater danger from psychiatric patients than from general medical patients
    (b) Fear rather than anger is a common cause of violence
    (c) Eye contact is useful in diffusing potentially violent situations
    (d) Giving instructions to the person will help to reduce the likelihood of violence
    (e) You should never see a person with a psychiatric history on your own

85 (a) **False**
   (b) **True**
   (c) **False**
   (d) **False**
   (e) **True**

The Mental State Examination is performed throughout the contact you have with the person. Unlike the physical examination it is not a separate entity to be performed once the history has been taken. All along you must be listening not only to what the person says, but also to the way in which they say it and their behaviour whilst saying it. This is not a difficult skill – just look and listen! The Mental State Examination describes only those experiences that the person is having at the time of the interview. If the person says that a week ago they heard voices of people they could not see, but not right now, this is part of the history, not the mental state. When discussing the mood of the person in the Mental State Examination you need to say something about the person's description of their mood (subjective) and your own assessment of it (objective). Biological features of depression help you to make a diagnosis of depressive episode or illness, but are part of the history, not the mental state. You cannot assume inner processes from a person's behaviour – you need to ask them why they did this or that: 'You appear to be listening for something. What can you hear?'

The surroundings a person finds themselves in are important and very useful to describe in the appearance and behaviour section of the mental state. Where you see someone, who was there and the nature of the surroundings can profoundly influence their behaviour.

86 (a) **False**
   (b) **True**
   (c) **False**
   (d) **False**
   (e) **False**

Generally speaking, people with a psychiatric history are unlikely to be violent. There are increasing numbers of attacks on medical staff in all disciplines, reflecting a more violent society. It is often the case that the people you see in acute situations are frightened and do not understand your intentions towards them, which gives rise to the violence. It is very threatening to make eye-to-eye contact for any length of time. It is better to avert your eyes and avoid confrontation. Similarly if people are offered choices or suggestions they are more likely to comply than if they are issued with instructions or orders, Always explain what you are doing and why. Try to seek answers to problems that you are both happy with. If you have any concerns about seeing a person with a history of psychiatric disorder make sure that you see them with someone and in a place where suitably trained staff are readily available.

87 Lithium: long-term adverse effects can be detected by monitoring:

    (a) Thyroid function (TFTs)
    (b) Creatinine clearance
    (c) Liver function (LFTs)
    (d) Serum calcium
    (e) Blood glucose level

88 Section 2 of the Mental Health Act 1983:

    (a) Requires the signatures of one doctor and one social worker
    (b) Permits compulsory admission and treatment for up to 6 months
    (c) Cannot be used to prevent promiscuous behaviour
    (d) Cannot be used to prevent elicit drug use
    (e) Is for the observation of the patient

87 **(a) True**
   (b) True
   (c) False
   (d) False
   (e) False

About 50 per cent of patients with bipolar affective disorder respond well to prophylactic lithium, whilst the rest show either a partial response or no response (Goodwin, F K. and Jameson, K. R. 1990: *Manic depressive illness*, Oxford: Oxford University Press). Carbamazepine appears to be about as effective as lithium in the prophylaxis of bipolar disorder. While the relapse rate of bipolar patients on maintenance placebo is over 80 per cent, the relapse rate on lithium is about 50 per cent while careful compliance with maintenance lithium significantly increases the remission rate above 50 per cent. Lithium prophylaxis is indicated for recurrent affective disorders with an interval of less than 2 or 3 years between episodes.

The important long-term side-effects of lithium therapy are the development of renal damage and of hypothyroidism. Regular monitoring of the serum lithium level helps to keep the drug within the range that will be both therapeutically effective and also reduce the likelihood of damage to the kidneys and thyroid gland Regular (3-monthly once established) monitoring is required. Creatinine clearance would be the best indication of developing renal damage but, in practice, regular serum creatinine estimations are the most useful index of renal functions in patients taking prophylactic lithium.

88 **(a) False**
   (b) False
   (c) True
   (d) True
   (e) False

Section 2 of the Mental Health Act 1983 allows the admission of a person who is suspected to be suffering from a mental disorder or severe mental impairment to hospital for 28 days in order that the person may be *assessed*. The enactment of the section requires the signatures of not only a qualified psychiatrist but also another doctor who has some previous knowledge of the person concerned (usually their GP), or if the GP is not available an independent but qualified psychiatrist. Once these two medical recommendations have been obtained, then a social worker with specific mental health training (an approved social worker ASW) can recommend that the section be enacted.

The section cannot be used to prevent promiscuity or illicit drug use.

89 Section 4 of the Mental Health Act 1983:

- (a) Cannot be used for persons over the age of 65 years
- (b) Can only be used for mentally disordered offenders
- (c) Can only be used in an emergency
- (d) Can only be used if children are at risk
- (e) Has to be implemented by two doctors and a social worker

90 Section 136 of the Mental Health Act 1983:

- (a) Authorizes the transfer of a person to a medium secure unit
- (b) Authorizes the transfer of a person to a 'place of safety'
- (c) Is implemented by an approved social worker (ASW)
- (d) Is implemented by the police
- (e) Is implemented by the hospital chaplain

89 **(a) False**
   (b) False
   (c) True
   (d) False
   (e) False

Section 4 of the Mental Health Act 1983 is a section allowing the admission of a person who is believed to be mentally ill to hospital for 72 h. It is only to be used in an emergency when an assessment for Section 2 of the Act would cause an unreasonable delay in the care of the person assessed. It can be completed by one doctor and an approved social worker (and in exceptional circumstances by the person's nearest relative). There are no stipulations of age, nor is it one of the battery of 'forensic' sections of the Act. If children are at risk then the normal provisions of the act apply, but steps to remove the children in the Children's Act 1990 may have to be taken.

90 **(a) False**
   (b) True
   (c) False
   (d) True
   (e) False

Section 136 of the Mental Health Act 1983 allows a police officer who has reason to believe a person *in a public place* is suffering from a mental disorder to remove that person to a 'place of safety' where an assessment of their mental state can take place. The section may lapse once the assessment has taken place. The section is for 72 h but in practice the assessment should take place within hours of arrival in the place of safety (very often an accident and emergency department). The assessment should be performed by a qualified psychiatrist and an approved social worker, and converted to a Section 2 if further assessment is required in hospital. The hospital chaplain has no formal role under the Mental Health Act, but his or her importance within the hospital, particularly to people with emotional disorders, should not be underestimated.

91 The Supervision Register is:

   (a) A list of paedophiles, kept at every police station
   (b) A list of schoolchildren excluded because of persistent disruptive behaviour
   (c) A list of people with psychiatric disorder who have a history of violent behaviour when unwell
   (d) A list of senior psychotherapists who instruct trainees
   (e) A list of all people who have been compulsorily detained under the Mental Health Act

92 Obsessive-compulsive disorder:

   (a) Is characterized by third-person auditory hallucinations
   (b) Typically includes arachnophobia
   (c) Includes a fear of uttering a blasphemy in church
   (d) Has a good prognosis if it occurs for the first time during an episode of severe depression
   (e) Is characterized by nihilistic delusions

91 **(a) False**
  (b) False
  (c) True
  (d) False
  (e) False

The Supervision Register is a list of people who suffer from severe psychiatric disorder who are at risk of:

(a) committing serious violence;
(b) suicide;
(c) severe self-neglect.

The aim of this register is to facilitate communication between professionals so that the complex needs of these people are met, one person is responsible for co-ordinating and regularly reviewing (with the multidisciplinary team) their care, and any early signs of relapse are picked up and acted upon. Information from the register should be available 24 h a day. Many of these people will have been detained under the Mental Health Act at some time or another, and will be subject to the provisions of Section 117 of the Act, which stipulate the need for care after discharge from Section 3 (6-month treatment order).

92 **(a) False**
  (b) False
  (c) True
  (d) True
  (e) False

The important features of obsessive-compulsive disorder are:

(a) thoughts or actions that come unbidden;
(b) thoughts or actions that are recognized as coming from 'within the person';
(c) thoughts or actions that are recognized as irrational.

The thoughts or actions often cannot be resisted, and the degree of resistance may vary from day to day and at different phases of the illness. It is not uncommon for the sufferer to fear uttering a blasphemy in church. The prognosis for the illness is much better if it occurs as part of a depressive illness than as a primary illness. Treatment may be with medication (especially high-dose selective serotonin reuptake inhibitors or SSRIs), but relapse is not uncommon once the medication is stopped. Psychological and behavioural approaches can also be undertaken. *If* the illness persists beyond 1 year the prognosis is poor.

Arachnophobia is a fear of spiders and is not a characteristic of OCD. The disorder also has no psychotic phenomena (delusions and hallucinations).

93 In closed head injury:

- (a) The amount of brain damage is directly proportional to the duration of retrograde amnesia
- (b) The long-term neuropsychological and occupational outcome is directly proportional to the duration of post-traumatic amnesia
- (c) Sensitivity to alcohol may ensue
- (d) Long-term memory is more severely affected than short-term memory
- (e) Complaints of lack of energy, irritability and poor concentration are highly suggestive of malingering

94 Anorexia nervosa:

- (a) Is never followed by bulimia
- (b) Is never fatal
- (c) Is associated with amenorrhoea
- (d) Is caused by pituitary cachexia
- (e) Is associated with a tendency to overestimate one's bodily dimensions

93 **(a) False**
    (b) True
    (c) True
    (d) False
    (e) False

The brain has been likened to a blancmange in a bowl. When it suffers closed injury, the blancmange twists and squashes up against the walls of the bowl. This causes not only contusions to the surface, but rotational injury to axons. There is diffuse damage due to shearing strains on the neurones, which cause them to stretch and tear. There is also stretching and tearing of small blood vessels causing oedema, compression and eventually ischaemia. This second subtle form of injury cannot be seen by current neuro-imaging techniques. People with head injuries may become more sensitive to any drug that acts directly upon the brain. This includes alcohol. Short-term memory is much more likely to suffer than long-term memory following closed head injury. In closed head injuries from road traffic accidents, the sub-frontal and anterior temporal regions suffer most from direct contusion, so that disturbances due to frontal and temporal damage might be added to the diffuse damage.

The 'Post-concussion syndrome' is relatively common following closed head injury (10–20 per cent of severe cases). The symptoms of fatigue, irritability and poor concentration sometimes with anxiety or depression, may take a long time to resolve. They may also be related to the pre-morbid nature of the person, and also to the meaning of the injury to them. This should be distinguished from malingering.

94 **(a) False**
    (b) False
    (c) True
    (d) False
    (e) True

Anorexia nervosa can be a fatal disorder. Mortality is 22 per cent higher than that expected for the general population of the same age, with two-thirds of deaths being due to the direct effects of the anorexia nervosa, and one-third due to suicide. Mortality is therefore significantly higher than for schizophrenia or bipolar affective disorder. Medical sequelae of long-term cases include stunted growth, sterility, renal failure and severe osteoporosis. The physical symptoms of anorexia nervosa are all secondary to starvation. It is estimated that there is a prevalence of between 1 and 2 per cent in female school children and university students. The sex ratio is of the order of 1 male to 20 females. The peak age of onset for anorexia nervosa is 17 years. The disorder occurs more commonly in social classes 1, 2 and 3.

When anorexia nervosa becomes life threatening because of very severe weight loss or severe depression with a risk of suicide, it may be necessary to admit the person for treatment under the Mental Health Act.

95 Bulimia nervosa:

   (a) Is characterized by bouts of bingeing
   (b) Is characterized by self-induced vomiting
   (c) Is characterized by very severe weight loss
   (d) Is characterized by purgative abuse
   (e) Is characterized by feelings of self-disgust

96 Phobias:

   (a) Social phobia is an irrational fear of the underclass
   (b) Simple phobias are much commoner in women than in men
   (c) Blood/injury phobia is accompanied by tachycardia
   (d) Phobias can respond well to treatment by behavioural methods that involve prolonged exposure
   (e) Xenophobia is treatable by SSRIs

95 (a) True
   (b) True
   (c) False
   (d) True
   (e) True

The characteristic features of bulimia nervosa, which was first described in 1979, are recurrent episodes of binge eating, recurrent attempts to prevent weight gain, including abuse of laxatives, diuretics and appetite suppressants, strict dieting, vigorous exercise and self-induced vomiting and a tendency to estimate one's value in terms of one's contours and weight. The bulimic patient Is usually within the normal weight range. Some patients with bulimia nervosa have hypertrophy of the parotid glands. In those who engage in self-induced vomiting there is erosion of the dental enamel. Menstruation tends to be irregular. Hypokalaemic alkalosis and raised serum amylase levels can be found. The most effective form of treatment is with cognitive behaviour therapy.

96 (a) False
   (b) False
   (c) False
   (d) True
   (e) False

The treatment of simple phobias is carried out by prolonged exposure to the phobic object or situation. Social phobias and agoraphobia respond best to a combination of prolonged exposure and cognitive techniques which are designed to eliminate 'fear of fear' and 'fear of negative evaluation' (see Hawton, K., Salkovskis, P. M., Kirk, J. W., and Clark, D. M. 1989: *Cognitive behavioural approaches for adult psychiatric disorders: a practical guide* Oxford: Oxford University Press). All phobias except blood/injury phobias are accompanied by the physiological response of arousal, which includes tachycardia.

97 Temporal lobe epilepsy is characterized by:

  (a) *Déjà vu*
  (b) *Jamais vu*
  (c) Olfactory hallucinations
  (d) Gustatory hallucinations
  (e) Cannot be provoked by severe anxiety

98 Neuroleptic malignant syndrome is characterized by:

  (a) Hypothermia
  (b) Muscle flaccidity
  (c) Elevated CPK
  (d) Occurrence only after administration of butyrophenones
  (e) Occurrence only after the administration of clozapine

97 (a) True
   (b) True
   (c) True
   (d) True
   (e) False

Partial seizures with complex symptoms generally arise in the temporal and frontal lobes. The symptoms include impairment of consciousness, autonomic effects, cognitive phenomena including amnesia, *déjà vu* and *jamais vu*, as well as disturbances of thinking and of speech, mood disturbance, perceptual disorders including illusions, hallucinations and depersonalization, and also automatism.

Temporal lobe epilepsy follows a characteristic pattern of fear and epigastric discomfort rising to the throat, to be followed rapidly by perceptual phenomena with hallucinations in any modality and a variety of transient emotional disturbances. Hallucinations of taste and smell may be accompanied by smacking of the lips or chewing movements. Any particular patient's sequence of events during the seizure tends to be replicated from fit to fit.

The diagnosis is essentially a clinical one, with the EEG often being normal.

98 (a) False
   (b) False
   (c) True
   (d) False
   (e) False

This is a rare and potentially fatal idiosyncratic reaction to antipsychotic therapy. The onset occurs after an interval of 2 to 28 days, and the clinical features include muscular rigidity, akinesia, high temperature, fluctuating levels of consciousness and hypertension and sweating. The patient may be incontinent. There is neutrophilia, elevated creatinine phosphokinase and raised potassium. The antipsychotic drug has to be withdrawn immediately and the patient admitted to a medical intensive care unit. Ominous developments include rhabdomyolysis, myoglobin anaemia and renal failure. Neuroleptic malignant syndrome can occur with any neuroleptic. In addition to the immediate withdrawal of all neuroleptics, management includes either Dantrolene or the dopamine antagonists, bromocriptine, L-dopa or apomorphine (Levenson, J. L., 1985: Neuroleptic malignant syndrome. *American Journal of Psychiatry* **142**, 1137–45).

99 Tardive dyskinesia is more likely to:

(a) Follow the use of depot rather than oral neuroleptics
(b) Only be caused by phenothiazines
(c) Be less likely to occur if the person has 'drug holidays'
(d) Possibly improve in the long term with cessation of the causative drug
(e) Possibly improve in the short term with an increase in the dose of the causative drug

99 (a) **False**
   (b) **False**
   (c) **False**
   (d) **True**
   (e) **True**

Tardive dyskinesia has an incidence of approximately 15 per cent in those taking neuroleptic medication. Risk factors include advanced age and the presence of affective disorder and organic brain disease. Orofacial and buccal-lingual involuntary movements and choreo-athetoid movements of the limbs can also occur.

The syndrome can also occur among normal elderly people, in people with schizophrenia who have not received any medication, and in the mentally impaired. Because of the risk of tardive dyskinesia, neuroleptic drugs should only be prescribed when absolutely necessary. Low-potency D_2 receptor blockers are preferable, and they should be given in the smallest possible doses.

Paradoxically, neuroleptic drugs can suppress tardive dyskinesia in the short term. 'Drug holidays' appear to increase the risk of tardive dyskinesia. While all of the typical neuroleptics might cause tardive dyskinesia, whether administered orally or as depot, there is some evidence that clozapine might have a therapeutic effect in tardive dyskinesia.

One theory for the development of tardive dyskinesia is that D_2 receptor blockade causes denervation, hypersensitivity and hyperdensity of D_2 receptors in the basal ganglia. Tardive dyskinesia can be made worse by anticholinergic medication, but it often appears if neuroleptic drugs are suddenly withdrawn.

The second most common type of tardive (late) syndrome is tardive dystonia, which consists of an involuntary contraction of the head and neck muscles. Clinical features are very similar to acute drug-induced dystonia, idiopathic torsion dystonia and secondary dystonia associated with Wilson's disease and Huntington's syndrome.

100 Post-traumatic stress disorder is characterized by:

- (a) 'Flashbacks' to one's childhood
- (b) Hypervigilance
- (c) Hypersomnolence
- (d) Hyperphagia
- (e) Hyperbole

100 (a) **False**
  (b) **True**
  (c) **False**
  (d) **False**
  (e) **False**

Prevalence rates for post-traumatic stress disorder (PTSD) can range from about 30 per cent among Australian firefighters (McFarlane, A. C. 1988: The longitudinal course of post-traumatic morbidity: the range of outcomes and their predictors. *Journal of Nervous and Mental Diseases* **176**, 30–40) to over 80 per cent among Cambodian refugees (Bernstein, C. E. and Rosser-Hogan, R. 1991: Trauma experiences, post-traumatic stress, dissociation and depression in Cambodian refugees. *American Journal of Psychiatry*, **148**, 1548–1). Predisposing factors for the development of PTSD after exposure to a life-threatening incident include neuroticism as a personality trait and a previous history of psychiatric disorder. In addition to these vulnerability factors, PTSD might be more likely to develop in those who are exposed to the greatest objective danger and threat to survival. PTSD is often accompanied by other disorders, notably alcohol dependence, atypical depression and pathological grief, and an anxiety disorder other than PTSD.

It is important to be aware of two other types of reaction to severe stress. An acute stress reaction is a transient disorder which develops in response to exceptional physical or mental stress. The onset occurs within a few minutes and the reaction usually subsides within about 3 days. Clinical features include a state of 'daze', with some constriction of the field of consciousness and narrowing of attention, impaired comprehension and disorientation. Associated symptoms include transient depression, anxiety, anger, despair, and agitation and over-activity or withdrawal. This condition is synonymous with 'psychic shock' and combat fatigue.

Adjustment disorders are states of distress and emotional disturbance which develop within 1 month of a stressful life event, and usually last no longer than a few months. The symptoms of adjustment disorder include lowering of mood, anxiety, worry, difficulty in coping or planning ahead, and some impairment of the ability to carry out normal daily activities. There is often a mixture of symptoms, but in themselves the symptoms are not sufficiently severe to justify a more specific diagnosis such as an anxiety state or a depressive disorder. A typical situation in which a person might develop an adjustment disorder would be on being informed by a doctor that they are suffering from cancer, or that they are HIV-positive.

101 Normal people:

- (a) Have delusions
- (b) Experience hallucinations
- (c) Have myoclonic jerks
- (d) Can be thought disordered
- (e) Have mood swings

101 **(a) False**
    (b) True
    (c) True
    (d) True
    (e) True

A delusional belief is one held with utter conviction despite evidence to the contrary, and that cannot be explained by the cultural, educational or social background of the person holding it. It is the product of pathological thought processes. Despite the fact that many people hold seemingly bizarre beliefs that seem to drive them and dominate their lives, they can usually be explained in terms of the person's background, and are not the result of pathological thought processes.

Hallucinations are relatively common in the normal population. Hearing your name called very clearly in a shop or at the railway station is common. Normal people in unusual circumstances, e.g. when widowed, over-tired (wait for your house jobs!) or in sensory deprivation will commonly experience hallucinations, and need reassurance that they are normal.

At times of great anxiety, e.g. vivas, our thoughts may not be expressed in their usual elegant lucid manner. Some people seem chronically unable to put together a coherent line of thought highly suggestive of the problems experienced by those with schizophrenia.

Myoclonic jerks happen as people drop off to sleep. They can be quite frightening but need no more than reassurance and an understanding partner. However, if they occur at other times they may be a sign of degenerative neurological disorder and require investigation.

Mood swings are part of everyday life. Most people's moods fluctuate within relatively narrow bands appropriate to the situation. For some people these bands are rather wider (cyclothymic personality disorder), and the moods seem to go in cycles. It is important to remember that people who have experienced a mental disorder continue to undergo fluctuations in mood, interest and volition just like everyone else, and this does not mean that relapse is imminent. These changes can cause great anxiety in families who are ever vigilant for signs of recurrence.

102 Features of somatization disorder include:

    (a) Bitter complaints about one particular part of the body
    (b) No physical basis demonstrated
    (c) Several weeks' duration
    (d) Onset generally in old age
    (e) The individual trying to avoid contact with the medical services
    (f) The individual altering their life-style as a result of their symptoms

103 Ecstasy:

    (a) Is a synthetic, heroin-like compound
    (b) Is a psychostimulant
    (c) Can cause fatal hyperthermia
    (d) Is MDMA
    (e) Can cause chronic paranoid psychosis

102 **(a) False**
   (b) True
   (c) False
   (d) False
   (e) False
   (f) True

In the detection of psychological disorders that present with somatic symptoms, the following information should be sought (Creed, F. H. 1992: Relationship of non-organic abdominal pain to psychiatric disorder and life stress. In Creed, F., Mayou, R. and Hopkins, A. (eds), *Medical symptoms not explained by organic disease.* London: Royal College of Psychiatrists and Royal College of Physicians, 9–16). Is a presenting bodily symptom accompanied by psychological symptoms or other physical symptoms typical of anxiety or depression? Is the somatic symptom typical of physical disorder? Has there been a previous episode of medically unexplained symptoms? Is the physical symptom triggered by stress and diminished by the relief of stress? Is there a family or personal history of psychiatric disorder? A trial of psychological treatment might relieve symptoms that have failed to respond to medical treatment.

The important features of somatization disorder are:

   (a) multiple complaints in several physical systems;
   (b) no physical basis demonstrated;
   (c) several years' duration;
   (d) Onset usually below 30 years of age;
   (e) frequent medical consultations;
   (f) the person changing their life-style because of the symptoms.

103 **(a) False**
   (b) True
   (c) True
   (d) True
   (e) True

Ecstasy is an amphetamine analogue MDMA, i.e. 3,4 methylenedioxy-methamphetamine. Like amphetamine, it has stimulant properties as well as being potentially cardiotoxic. Its use has been associated with deaths from hyperthermia, especially at 'raves'. Like amphetamine, it can cause chronic paranoid psychosis. MDA which is 3,4 methylenedioxyamphetamine has the additional toxic property in primates of destroying central serotonergic terminals.

104 Abnormal movements:

   (a) Mannerisms are abnormal, repetitive, non-goal-directed movements

   (b) A tic is a sudden, involuntary twitching of groups of muscles, especially in the face

   (c) Stereotypies are regular, repetitive, goal-directed movements or utterances

   (d) Spasmodic torticollis consists of twisting of the head due to spasm of the neck muscles

   (e) In echopraxia, the person imitates the movement of the interviewer

104 **(a) False**
    (b) True
    (c) False
    (d) True
    (e) True

Abnormal movements can be classified as (a) disorders of adaptive movement, e.g. mannerisms, and (b) non-adaptive movements which can be divided into spontaneous movements, including tics, spasmodic torticollis and stereotypies, and induced movements, including echopraxia.

Mannerisms are abnormal, repetitive, goal-directed movements such as a bizarre style of walking, as in chronic schizophrenia. A mannerism is an apparently purposeful act which is consistently carried out in an odd or unusual way.

Tics are stereotyped, irregularly repetitive jerking movements of a single muscle group, especially in the face. The patient is aware of them. They are common and usually remit in childhood. They can occur when associated with tension in adults, and can also be drug-induced and might follow trauma or encephalitis. In a severe form they are seen in Gilles de la Tourette's syndrome.

Stereotypies are regular, repetitive stereotyped non-goal-directed movements such as rocking of the body. Stereotyped utterances can occur. These abnormal movements can be seen in chronic schizophrenia and in severe learning disabilities.

Spasmodic torticollis, like blepharospasm, is a variety of focal dystonia which is thought to have an organic basis. Tardive dystonia can occur after prolonged use of neuroleptics.

Echopraxia is the spontaneous copying of another person's movements or gestures. Other examples of induced movements include automatic obedience, echolalia (the imitation of words or phrases), perseveration (the senseless repetition of a previously requested movement), and mitgehen (in which slight pressure leads to movement in any direction, although the subject is being asked to resist).

(See Hamilton, M. (ed.), 1974: *Fish's clinical psychopathology*. Bristol: Wright).

105 Hallucinations:

- (a) A pseudohallucination is located in external space
- (b) Functional hallucinations are experienced along with a background stimulus
- (c) Hypnagogic hallucinations occur in normal people while falling asleep
- (d) Lilliputian hallucinations do not suggest an organic state
- (e) Musical hallucinations can occur in temporal lobe epilepsy
- (f) Elementary hallucinations are suggestive of epilepsy

105 (a) False
   (b) True
   (c) True
   (d) False
   (e) True
   (f) True

In 1833, Esquirol defined hallucinations as perceptions which arise in the absence of any external stimulus. Pseudohallucinations are experienced as originating from within the mind, and they are located in subjective rather than objective space. Pseudohallucinations lack the substantiality of real perceptions. They differ from a vivid mental image in that there is no voluntary control over pseudohallucinations, i.e. they cannot be conjured up deliberately.

Functional hallucinations are provoked by a stimulus and are experienced along with that stimulus, e.g. hearing voices in the sound of a motor car engine. Hypnagogic and hypnopompic (occurring while waking up) hallucinations occur in normal people. They may be visual or auditory.

In Lilliputian hallucinations (micropsia) objects hallucinated are seen as smaller than they would appear if real, e.g. the person sees miniature people. Lilliputian hallucinations can occur in temporal lobe epilepsy, drug use, delirium tremens and disorders of the eye. The commonest cause is an acute organic state such as delirium tremens.

Elementary hallucinations include tingling, light flashes and buzzing, and are suggestive of epilepsy. An occipital lobe focus might produce flashes of light or zig-zag patterns.

106 The expression of emotion:

(a) Cyclothymia is a tendency to experience pronounced swings of mood from cheerful to unhappy
(b) Rapid cycling is a tendency to drive recklessly in hypomania and mania
(c) Emotional incontinence is loss of control over the emotions with rapid fluctuations, seen in organic disorders
(d) Anhedonia is the inability to feel pleasure
(e) Hyperthymia is a tendency to be unrealistically sad, miserable and despondent

106 **(a) True**
    (b) False
    (c) True
    (d) True
    (e) False

Cyclothymia is a tendency to experience marked fluctuations in mood, from cheerful to unhappy, often without clear precipitants for the changes. Whilst these fluctuations are obvious and clear, they are not severe enough to be called an illness.

Rapid cycling is a term used for those who have bipolar affective disorder which fluctuates rapidly from depression to mania and back again. It is probable that carbamazepine is a better prophylactic agent than lithium for those who experience this type of illness. Tricyclic antidepressants have been implicated in pushing people into rapid cycling, but this is a relatively rare occurrence, and the mechanism is not known.

Emotional incontinence is a loss of control over the emotion which is usually seen in those who have organic brain damage. It is common in dementing illness and can cause great distress to carers, whilst it is only very transient for the affected person. Tricyclic antidepressants can alleviate this symptom.

Anhedonia is an inability to experience pleasure, commonly reported by those who experience depressive illness.

Hyperthymia is the tendency to be cheerful almost whatever the circumstances, often to an irritating degree when everyone else is completely fed up with a situation! It does not reach the extremes of manic mood and is not an illness.

(Goodwin, F. K. and Jamison, K. R. 1990 *Manic-depressive Illness*. Oxford: Oxford University Press).

107 Chronic fatigue syndrome (CFS):

   (a) The population point prevalence for CFS is 2.6 per cent
   (b) Approximately one-tenth of patients with chronic CFS fulfil the criteria for affective disorder
   (c) Over one half of patients with Epstein-Barr virus infection develop CFS
   (d) Psychiatric disorders are no more common in CFS than in other physical illnesses such as rheumatoid arthritis
   (e) Structural and functional neuro-imaging have failed to show consistent abnormalities in CFS

107 (a) True
    (b) False
    (c) False
    (d) False
    (e) True

The 1996 report of the Royal Colleges of Physicians, Psychiatrists and General Practitioners on CFS states that the population point prevalence of CFS is 2.6 per cent in primary care. Up to 60 per cent of primary care or community cases of CFS fulfil the criteria for common psychological disorders – most frequently affective disorder, but there are also many cases of anxiety and somatization disorder. The depression found in 50 per cent of CFS patients is not merely secondary to the disability and uncertainty associated with CFS. Psychiatric disorders are much commoner in CFS than psychological disorders in other physical illnesses such as rheumatoid arthritis or multiple sclerosis.

Structural and functional neuro-imaging and neuroendocrinological investigations have not led to consistent abnormalities being demonstrated in CFS, and there is no compelling evidence for a primary role of neuromuscular dysfunction. Reports of cognitive abnormalities are inconsistent, and are confounded by sleep disturbance and mood disorder. There is no consistent evidence of primary disorder of muscle structure or function in CFS, and there is no convincing evidence that common viral infections are a risk factor for CFS, except for infection with the Epstein-Barr virus. However, less than 10 per cent of those with Epstein-Barr virus develop CFS. The evidence for disturbance of immune function as a primary aetiological factor in CFS is currently weak. Previous personality factors and psychological distress appear to be more important than common viral infections, both in terms of causation and in perpetuating disability. There are no laboratory tests that establish or confirm a diagnosis of CFS. Laboratory investigation to exclude an alternative physical diagnosis should be limited to full blood count, ESR, liver function tests, urea and electrolytes, TSH and free thyroxine, creatine kinase and urine analysis for protein and sugar. The most effective form of treatment is graded exercise and/or cognitive behavioural therapy. There is no convincing evidence that any of the following treatments are effective: complementary therapy, dietary intervention, immunoglobulins, antihistamines, antiviral agents, magnesium or evening primrose oil. Antidepressants have a role in those patients with CFS and depressive disorders.

108 Epidemiology of Schizophrenia:

   (a) The lifetime risk of schizophrenia is approximately 0.1 per cent

   (b) In males the median age of onset of schizophrenia is 15 years earlier than in females

   (c) Paternal occupation displayed on birth certificates shows a disproportionate number of social class 4 and 5 occupations

   (d) There is an increased prevalence of left-handedness

   (e) There is an increased incidence of perinatal injury

109 Depression and social factors – in a study of depression in women in Camberwell, the sociologists Brown and Harris found:

   (a) An excess of childlessness

   (b) An excess of working mothers

   (c) An excess of threatening life events or long-term difficulties such as poor housing

   (d) Lack of a confiding relationship

   (e) Loss of mother before the age of 11 years

108 (a) **False**
   (b) **False**
   (c) **False**
   (d) **True**
   (e) **True**

The lifetime risk of schizophrenia is approximately 1 per cent, with an incidence of 15 to 20 per 100 000 population per year. The usual age of onset is 15 to 45 years, and in males the onset is 5 years earlier than in females. The occupations of fathers of patients with schizophrenia show the same class distribution as the general population, so the increased prevalence in deprived inner-city areas is. mainly due to downward social drift. There is an increased prevalence of left-handedness and an increased incidence of perinatal injury. Patients with schizo-phrenia are more often single and show low fertility. 'Soft' neurological signs such as astereognosis, clumsiness and abnormality of gait are found in many patients with chronic schizophrenia, even if they have received very little drug treatment. Neurological 'soft' signs occur in up to 60 per cent of patients with schizophrenia, but there is no specific abnormality.

109 (a) **False**
   (b) **False**
   (c) **True**
   (d) **True**
   (e) **True**

Brown and Harris (Brown, G. and Harris, T. 1978: *Social origins of depression.* London: Tavistock) attributed depression in women in south London to a combination of provoking agents, such as major adverse life events and long-term problems, together with vulnerability factors which included:

  (a) no employment outside the home;
  (b) lack of a confiding relationship;
  (c) three or more children under the age of 14 years at home;
  (d) loss of mother before the age of 11 years.

Working-class women had higher rates of depression and experienced more vulnerability factors than middle-class women.

110 Clozapine:

    (a) Acts by D_2 receptor blockade
    (b) Can cause agranulocytosis in up to 2 per cent of people
    (c) Can be effective in treatment-refractory schizophrenia
    (d) Rarely causes extrapyramidal side-effects
    (e) Can cause grand mal seizures

111 Family interaction and schizophrenia – patients with schizophrenia are more vulnerable to psychotic relapse if they live with relatives who:

    (a) Are detached
    (b) Are hostile
    (c) Are critical
    (d) Spend more than 35 h per week with the patient in a setting of high expressed emotion (EE)
    (e) Are tolerant

112 Fugues can occur:

    (a) After head injury
    (b) After a seizure
    (c) During a depressive illness
    (d) In a dissociative state
    (e) In Gilles de la Tourette's syndrome

110 **(a) False**
  (b) True
  (c) True
  (d) True
  (e) True

Clozapine is an 'atypical' antipsychotic drug which can be effective in at least one-third of people with schizophrenia who have failed to respond to other classes of antipsychotic medication. It has a low occupancy of D_2 receptors and it may act via D_4 receptors. Because of the risk of agranulocytosis, which can occur in up to 2 per cent of people taking the drug, regular and frequent blood tests are mandatory. Clozapine is withdrawn if there is a decrease in white cells or if the person fails to comply with regular blood tests. Most cases of agranulocytosis have occurred within the first 6 months of treatment, with a gradual mode of onset. The commonest adverse reactions to clozapine are drowsiness, hyper-salivation and tachycardia. Clozapine, like other antipsychotic drugs, lowers the seizure threshold leading to grand mal seizures. Extrapyramidal side-effects are minimal.

111 **(a) False**
  (b) True
  (c) True
  (d) True
  (e) False

People with schizophrenia who live in a home with relatives who are critical, hostile and over-involved, i.e. who are high on expressed emotion (EE), are more vulnerable to psychotic relapse. People living with families with high expressed emotion derive additional protective benefit from antipsychotic drugs compared with people living in more tolerant environments. Training the family to reduce expressed emotion and educating close relatives about schizophrenia can reduce the rate of relapse.

112 **(a) True**
  (b) True
  (c) True
  (d) True
  (e) False

A fugue is characterized by wandering from the person's usual surroundings with superficially normal behaviour. There is amnesia for the episode, and occasionally a new identity is assumed.

Post-epileptic fugues are less purposeful and there is evidence of a confusional state. Other organic causes of wandering include dementia, acute confusional states including hypoglycaemic episodes, black-outs and alcoholism and head injury. Psychogenic causes include depression, an acute reaction to overwhelming stress, and malingering.

113 Munchausen's syndrome:

    (a) Is a fictitious disorder
    (b) Is a factitious disorder
    (c) Is commoner in women
    (d) Has abdominal symptoms as the commonest presenting complaint
    (e) Might present with false bereavements

114 Alcoholic hallucinosis:

    (a) Is accompanied by little or no clouding of consciousness
    (b) Is characterized by third-person auditory hallucinations
    (c) Is accompanied by bizarre 'non-understandable' delusions
    (d) About one-fifth of cases are eventually diagnosed as suffering from schizophrenia
    (e) Does not have a clear temporal link with alcohol withdrawal

115 Tic disorders:

    (a) Reduce during sleep
    (b) Are associated with demonstrable neurological abnormality
    (c) In Tourette's syndrome are accompanied by involuntary explosive obscene utterances
    (d) Haloperidol in low doses can significantly reduce tics in most cases
    (e) May be associated with abnormalities in the mid-brain dopaminergic system

113 (a) **False**
   (b) **True**
   (c) **False**
   (d) **True**
   (e) **True**

Munchausen's syndrome is a term coined by Richard Asher, a general physician, in 1951, to describe people who simulate symptoms of acute disease in order to gain admission to hospital (it is also known as hospital addiction syndrome). The person, often an itinerant male using an alias, most commonly presents with abdominal symptoms but haematemesis, chest pain and renal colic are not infrequent. Once in hospital, the person may develop new symptoms when investigation of the original symptom is negative. The course tends to be chronic with multiple admissions.

114 (a) **True**
   (b) **True**
   (c) **False**
   (d) **True**
   (e) **True**

Alcoholic hallucinosis consists of auditory hallucinations in the third person occurring in clear consciousness. The hallucinations are derogatory or menacing. They might be accompanied by secondary delusions which attempt to explain the voices. The condition may occur during a bout of heavy drinking or on withdrawal. Recovery is usually within weeks or months of giving up alcohol completely, but a small number of cases develop a chronic hallucinating illness. It is a differential diagnosis of schizophrenia, and about 20 per cent of cases go on to develop full-blown schizophrenia.

115 (a) **True**
   (b) **False**
   (c) **True**
   (d) **True**
   (e) **True**

A tic is a rapid, sudden, purposeless movement of a functionally related group of muscles, most commonly facial. In Gilles de la Tourette's syndrome, there are also vocal tics which appear as grunts and coprolalia (obscene utterances). Tics increase with anxiety and disappear during sleep. The onset is in childhood and adolescence. Boys are affected three times more often than girls. In the absence of Gilles de la Tourette's syndrome the prognosis is generally good. Haloperidol in doses of 2 to 3 mg daily is effective in most cases. However, since tic disorders can wax and wane, haloperidol should only be considered where the tic is established or where it is causing distress, e.g. as a result of teasing. Behavioural methods should be tried first.

116 Fetal alcohol syndrome includes:

    (a) Prenatal and/or postnatal growth retardation
    (b) Normal developmental milestones
    (c) Normal intellectual development
    (d) Mid-facial hypoplasia
    (e) Low birth weight but 'catch-up' growth

117 Systemic lupus erythematosus (SLE):

    (a) In SLE the central nervous system is affected in less than 50 per cent of cases
    (b) SLE can cause seizures
    (c) The commonest organic state associated with SLE is an acute organic reaction (delirium)
    (d) Clinical features include skin changes, renal damage and arthritis
    (e) Schizophreniform psychosis is common in SLE

118 Head injury prognosis – the outlook for neurological and psychosocial recovery is significantly worse:

    (a) With a duration of post-traumatic amnesia (PTA) longer than 24 h
    (b) With a penetrating head injury
    (c) With intracranial bleeding
    (d) With damage to the right parietal or right temporal lobe
    (e) In younger age groups

116 (a) True
    (b) False
    (c) False
    (d) True
    (e) False

Fetal alcohol syndrome occurs in the children of chronic alcoholic mothers. It is characterized by:

(a) low birth weight;
(b) retardation of postnatal growth;
(c) developmental delay;
(d) intellectual impairment;
(e) a characteristic faces with maxillary hypoplasia, small palpebral fissures and a poorly developed philtrum.

There is often mild to moderate mental retardation.

117 (a) False
    (b) True
    (c) True
    (d) True
    (e) False

In SLE, vasculitis causes multiple micro-infarcts. The central nervous system (CNS) is affected in 60 to 75 per cent of cases. People may also display psychiatric reactions to the steroids they are given to treat the SLE. The disturbances tend to be transient and fluctuating. Acute organic reactions (delirium) occur in up to 30 per cent of cases. Neurotic symptoms are common. Other conditions associated with SLE are dementia, depressive psychoses and, rarely, schizophreniform illness.

118 (a) True
    (b) True
    (c) True
    (d) False
    (e) False

The duration of PTA is defined as the length of time between the head injury and the restoration of clear and continuous memory. A poor prognosis following head injury is associated with long duration of impaired consciousness, a PTA of over 24 hs, and penetrating injury which carries a risk of epilepsy in up to 30 per cent of cases, combined with the possible psychiatric sequelae of epilepsy. The risk of permanent cognitive impairment increases with age. Personality change almost always occurs when there is severe intellectual impairment.

119 Medical aspects of alcohol abuse –1

    (a) About 20 per cent of men admitted to general medical wards are problem drinkers

    (b) In 20 per cent of road traffic accident fatalities, at least one of those involved has a blood alcohol concentration of over 80 mg %

    (c) Steady daily drinking of 6 units of alcohol for men and 3 units for women over a period of 10 years significantly increases the risk of developing cirrhosis

    (d) Good diet prevents the development of alcoholic cirrhosis

    (e) There is a 50 per cent mortality rate after 5 years from the time of diagnosis in patients with alcoholic cirrhosis who continue to consume alcohol

120 Medical aspects of alcohol abuse – 2

    (a) Excessive alcohol consumption is the main cause of chronic pancreatitis

    (b) Alcoholic cerebellar atrophy is largely irreversible

    (c) Alcohol is not a risk factor for the development of psoriasis

    (d) Avascular necrosis can be a complication of alcoholism

    (e) Heavy drinking causes prolongation of the QT interval on the ECG

119 **(a) True**
   (b) True
   (c) True
   (d) False
   (e) True

About one-fifth of men and one-tenth of women admitted to general hospitals are problem drinkers. One-tenth of non-fatal casualties occur in drink-drive accidents. While a good diet does not prevent the development of cirrhosis, poor nutrition exacerbates hepatic damage, as does previous viral hepatitis.

It is suggested that 14 units of alcohol (half a pint of beer, a glass of wine or a single measure of spirits) per week for a woman and 21 units per week for a man are 'safe' limits for alcohol consumption.

120 **(a) True**
   (b) True
   (c) False
   (d) True
   (e) True

Excessive alcohol consumption is involved in the aetiology of up to 85 per cent of chronic pancreatitis.

Alcoholic cerebellar atrophy is irreversible, unlike peripheral neuropathy, which improves with thiamine. However, the thiamine supplements do not prevent worsening of peripheral neuropathy if the patient continues to drink. Peripheral neuropathy occurs in about 10 per cent of very heavy drinkers.

Heavy drinking is associated with hypertension and strokes. All doctors should be alert for the features of the alcohol dependence syndrome (Edwards, G. and Gross, M. 1976: Alcohol dependence: provisional description of a clinical syndrome. *British Medical Journal* 1, 1058–61) which include:

   (a) a fixed drinking routine;
   (b) increased tolerance;
   (c) repeated withdrawal symptoms;
   (d) drinking to avoid or relieve withdrawal symptoms;
   (e) compulsion to drink and craving;
   (f) reinstatement after abstinence.

121 Psychiatric drugs and general medicine:

- (a) In epilepsy the antidepressant of first choice is a reversible inhibitor of monoaminoxidase – A (RIMA)
- (b) Fluoxetine (Prozac) can alter the serum level of anticonvulsants
- (c) Salbutamol can precipitate anxiety and agitation
- (d) Non-steroidal anti-inflammatory drugs can precipitate depression
- (e) There is no need to adjust the dose of anticoagulants when these are prescribed in combination with an SSRI

122 Huntington's disease:

- (a) Presents clinically in childhood
- (b) Is due to progressive atrophy of the lenticular nucleus
- (c) Is associated with sub-cortical dementia
- (d) The defective gene is located on the short arm of chromosome 4
- (e) Is characterized by choreiform movements

121 (a) **True**
    (b) **True**
    (c) **True**
    (d) **True**
    (e) **False**

People with organic brain syndromes and the elderly are especially susceptible to tricyclic antidepressants (e.g. dothiepin, imipramine) with strong anticholinergic side-effects, and up to 15 per cent of users may develop delirium. SSRIs which are free of anticholinergic effects are the antidepressant of choice in such cases.

Tricyclic antidepressants should be avoided by people with cardiovascular disorders as they can cause cardiac arrhythmias by increasing myocardial adrenaline levels, and by their anti-cholinergic and quinidine-like effects. They also depress myocardial contractility. SSRIs are the antidepressants of choice in cardiovascular disease. Tricyclic antidepressants are the first choice in renal disease. Both SSRIs and tricyclic antidepressants should be administered at a low dosage in liver disease.

Tricyclic antidepressants are preferable to SSRIs in diabetes.

In epilepsy, a RIMA or an SSRI is preferable to tricyclics, since the latter lower the seizure threshold (see 1996: Treatment methods and their effectiveness. In Guthrie, E. and Creed, F. (eds), *Seminars in liaison psychiatry*. London: Gaskell).

122 (a) **False**
    (b) **False**
    (c) **True**
    (d) **True**
    (e) **True**

Huntington's disease is characterized by:

    (a) choreiform movements;
    (b) dementia;
    (c) changes in behaviour, mood and personality.

The condition is inherited as an autosomal dominant and the defective gene is located on the short arm of chromosome 4. The neuropathology is progressive atrophy of the neostriatum, especially of the caudate nucleus, and there is excessive dopamine transmission. The onset is generally in middle age.

123 Psychotropic drugs and general medicine:

    (a) Pimozide can cause ventricular arrhythmias
    (b) Tricyclic antidepressants are contraindicated in renal failure
    (c) Antimuscarinic drugs are contraindicated in diabetes mellitus
    (d) Tricyclic antidepressants lower the seizure threshold
    (e) Lithium is contraindicated in liver disease

124 Phobic disorders:

    (a) Over 60 per cent of agoraphobic patients are female
    (b) Illness phobia is commoner in women than in men
    (c) Animal phobia is often accompanied by non-phobic psychiatric symptoms
    (d) Agoraphobia is often precipitated by major adverse life events
    (e) Social phobia is based on a fear of being exposed to the scrutiny of others

123 **(a) True**
   (b) False
   (c) False
   (d) True
   (e) False

Pimozide can cause prolonged QT interval, T-wave changes, ventricular arrhythmias and sudden death. An ECG before starting treatment is mandatory, and treatment should be started with low doses.

Whereas lower doses of all neuroleptics should be used because of increased cerebral sensitivity in renal impairment, tricyclic antidepressants can be given at normal doses. Antimuscarinics must be given with caution; whereas lithium is, of course, absolutely contraindicated in severe renal impairment.

Fluoxetine might cause hypoglycaemia in diabetics. There are no problems with antimuscarinic agents.

The sedative phenothiazines (chlorpromazine and promazine) lower the seizure threshold. Clozapine can also cause seizures with the risk increasing significantly at doses above 600 mg daily. All of the tricyclics lower the seizure threshold, especially amitriptyline. The SSRIs, RIMAs and MAOIs carry little risk of inducing convulsions. Fluphenazine, pimozide and sulpiride are claimed to have little epileptogenic effect.

Lithium is not contraindicated in liver disease. The high-risk psychotropic drugs in liver disease include lofepramine, MAOIs, and long-acting benzodiazepines in high doses. Sulpiride is safe with liver disease, but there is some risk associated with the use of phenothiazines, clozapine, risperidone and SSRIs, RIMAs and tricyclics.

124 **(a) True**
   (b) False
   (c) False
   (d) True
   (e) True

Agoraphobia is the commonest phobic disorder encountered in clinical practice. The majority of patients are female, with an onset before age 35 years of age. Strictly speaking, the term means 'fear of the market-place', but it is used to refer to fear and avoidance of open spaces as well as of enclosed or crowded spaces. It is often accompanied by generalized anxiety, panic attacks, depression, depersonalization and derealization. There is frequently a history of childhood fears and of precipitation of the agoraphobia by a major adverse life event. Social phobias are somewhat commoner in women. They develop in adolescence and early adulthood, and consist of a fear of behaving in a publicly embarrassing manner, together with a fear and avoidance of being exposed to the scrutiny of other people. Animal and other specific phobias are not generally accompanied by other psychiatric symptoms. Illness phobia occurs equally frequently in men and women, and may be precipitated by physical illness in the patient or a relative.